ACKNOWLEDGMENTS

MRS. OLIVE BROWN
For typing up, punctuating and spell-checking my handwritten account, then digitalising it. My eternal thanks Ollie.

TIM CARROLL
For kind permission to reproduce his portrait of me of 5th October 2010.

MESSRS. TONY HILLIER, MO NEEDHAM AND MATT HOLLAND
(Artswords worker, a Literature Development project for Swindon Borough Council)
For encouragement, advice and assistance in bringing the project to a conclusion. Without their assistance this would have remained a file of double-spaced typed paper on a bookshelf in my home.

JILL SHARP
For her efforts to encourage me in life writing. Although in order to do justice to Jill, I must admit I could not break the habit of a lifetime. I write as I speak – from the heart, giving the facts with little embellishment and NO fiction!

THE SWINDON ADVERTISER
Newspaper articles and pictures reproduced with the kind permission of the *Swindon Advertiser* Editor.

CONTENTS

Wartime and Immediate Post War Childhood

This story begins with the marriage of a heavy goods vehicle driver, by name Leonard F.G. Huzzey, and a seamstress, Ellen Sophia Jago (known as Nell) in Peckham, London SE15, on the 28th March 1937. In July 1938 Nell, as she was known to all, gave birth to their first child christened Anthony, reputedly after Anthony Eden although Len was a convinced Labour supporter!! Henceforth his son, alias myself, was known to all as Tony.

When, my mother, Nell fell pregnant with their second child my parents became tenants of the house next door to my father's parents at 218 Cator Street. This was a road of two-storey terraced late Victorian dwellings some half a mile in length bisected by two roads running east and west into three sections. This house, number 218, was located at the southern end of Cator Street some fifteen houses away from the first bisecting road.

Following the outbreak of war in September 1939 the transport firm for which my father worked came under government control and he, as a skilled HGV driver and also a father, was exempted from military service. My sister, Colleen, was born in August 1940.

One night, in either late 1940 or early 1941, a German bomber flew over the area possibly aiming for the Surrey Docks or the head of the Surrey Union Canal where a timber yard was set alight and roads of housing parallel to the canal were destroyed. In Cator Street the first seven houses down from the bisecting road above 218 took a direct hit and were completely destroyed with 218 suffering considerable blast damage. At the time myself, Colleen and our parents were fortunately ensconced in my paternal grandfather's Anderson shelter. He was a Boer War and First World War veteran and which his old Regimental Sergeant Major's (R.S.M.) experience of the trenches in the 1914-18 conflict, had, with my father's help dug his Anderson shelter very deep. This was covered with at least three feet of soil above its corrugated iron roof with enough space to accommodate the whole family including both my parents, myself and Colleen, still a baby, my father's two sisters, younger brother and both of his parents.

In the middle section of Cator Street, as revealed to myself when, as an eight year old I began exploring my surroundings, approximately twenty houses were missing and the school in the centre of that stretch of buildings had sustained considerable blast damage. In the bottom section a church had also suffered blast damage and houses adjacent to the canal had been completely destroyed.

Following the raid my father, his brother and my mother's cousins salvaged what they could from number 218 with their wedding photographs, Colleen's clothes and nappies, etc., being my mother's priorities. My puppy, Prince, which was my second year birthday present, was miraculously found alive having been sheltered between the keyboard and the top of my father's upright piano which had been knocked over by the blast. The puppy had been acquired because, as a toddler, I had become firmly attached to and established as a great playmate and friend of my maternal grandmother's black mongrel, a friendly, loping, harmless and tolerant animal with, in those un-politically correct days, the inevitable name of "nigger".

With our home rendered uninhabitable and with the inevitability of further bombing, my father loaded the family into the cab of his truck. This was not an easy task as the engines of the Scammell or Foden trucks occupied the centre of the cab and were situated between the seats of the driver and trailer mate. These vehicles, aside from the heat of the engine, were extremely cold and draughty. They also had no power steering or syncromesh, there was no such thing as automatic gearboxes and their brakes operated with only mini-mal ability. With a wagon and trailer, sometimes two, the loaded unit would be in excess of fifty tonnes. Journeys had to be undertaken with no road light-ing and only the "cats' eyes" in the centre of the main trunk roads to navigate by. Drivers of these rigs, apart from good eyesight, needed steady nerves, great concentration and tremendous strength which could be sustained over eight to twelve hours of continuous driving. In later years I became used to hearing my father described as being "built like a brick shit house, with the heart of a lion yet tender as a lamb".

The journey the family made was on one of my father's regular trunk runs to Stroud in Gloucestershire with my mother and we two children being delivered into the home of one of my father's friends at the Stroud depot. Saying farewell to his family my father then continued westward to the load's final destination in Cornwall.

Some months later, with the Luftwaffe now diverting its attentions more onto the ports and larger industrial centres, and following heavy raids in Bris-tol and the surrounding area, once again my mother and we two children were placed in the cab of my father's lorry and this time dropped off in Exeter at the house of Mr and Mrs Hardwick and their three teenage children, Gordon, Rita and Peggy. Their house was located on the outskirts of Exeter, opposite

DEDICATION

This book is dedicated to the memory of my late wife Joan, whose love, support and companionship, together with a great family and home life, made me determined that diabetes was not going to threaten its existence or continuance. It is to Joan I owe reason for my living for 61 years with the condition known as Type 1 Diabetes.

FOREWORD

After surviving the whole of the Second World War as a young child I was struck down with Type 1 Diabetes in 1950 at the age of 12. I nearly died, my weight dropped down to only 26 pounds but, thankfully, a doctor with the same condition helped me through. I have lived the last 61 years with diabetes and it hasn't beaten me yet!

I have attempted, in recounting my own experiences, to prove to all who may doubt it that a socially useful, personally fulfilling and thoroughly satisfactory and enjoyable life is possible with the chronic condition known at Type 1 Diabetes. My aim is to encourage those of you with the condition, or who are related to someone who has it, to do the same. Don't despair! Be resolute. If I can do it so, with the help and guidance I hope you'll find in my story, can you! Do as I did; don't allow it to stand in your way. You too can master it – *Go for it!*

to where green fields gave rise to low hills.

Some while after arriving in Exeter both Colleen and myself caught measles which subsequently led to scarlet fever resulting in us being admitted to hospital. Around this time, at the height of the blitz, my mother's younger, engaged sister, Daisy, and their youngest cousin Terry, who was ten, were also taken down to Exeter and accommodated at a house along the road. They all remained in Exeter which was where I started school.

On one occasion, when all the children were in the playground, a single-seater German aircraft swooped low over the area hotly pursued by what, to this day, I am convinced was a spitfire. Fortunately neither plane was firing its guns as they swept over the playground but very soon afterwards all the children scampered back into the school when actual gunfire was heard. This was rapidly followed by a distant explosion and through the classroom windows we could all see a rising column of smoke.

For some years after the war I experienced a recurring dream where I saw myself, together with my mother pushing my sister in a pushchair along a street on our way to visit the barbers, being pursued by a glass airplane in which the crew could clearly be seen.

In 1943 the Luftwaffe again changed tactics and following the so-called Baedeker raid on Exeter, the sisters, in view of Daisy's forthcoming marriage to her fiancée, Bert, a sergeant in the East Kents, decided that if they were going to be bombed they would rather be in London with their parents. Not being very happy with this idea, my father arranged for my mother and their two children to be housed in Reigate, outside London, for Daisy's wedding.

Someone had managed to acquire enough material to make an RAF uniform for myself, who was to be a pageboy, with one of Bert's nieces as a bridesmaid. On the wedding day, both us children, being about five or six years old at the time, were subsequently dressed and ready. We, however, made our way to the small rear garden where Daisy's father kept rabbits to supplement the family's meat ration. He had been painting the rabbit hutches some time before and had left the paintbrush in what little remained of the paint. Obviously with children being children, I promptly retrieved the paintbrush and daubed the bridesmaid who likewise retaliated. Luckily this incident did not subsequently appear to affect the relationship that either of us had with our uncle and aunt who would sometimes remind us of how we had nearly ruined their wedding day but this was always said with a grin on their respective faces.

At the start of the doodle bug bombing, with many of these initially falling short of their London target on the outskirts, my mother and us children returned to Furley Road. As we arrived and turned into Furley Road, some

250 yards from our grandparents' house, a large black dog accompanied by a smaller black and white one, came bounding down the street both barking excitedly. The smaller of the two took the lead and immediately leapt up striking me in the chest. I somehow managed to retain my balance and bent down towards the dog, my Prince, who eagerly began to lick my face. We had not seen each other for four years yet my grandmother assured me that both dogs had been barking and scratching at the front door to be let out for some minutes prior to the family's arrival.

Furley Road had been provided with a number of brick built shelters placed in the centre of the road. At the southern end, on the right hand side, all the houses which had been destroyed in the blitz had been replaced by a static water tank for the use of the Auxiliary Fire Service (A.F.S.). With the doodle bugs now striking Central London and the occasional bomber raid, nights were spent in one of the street shelters which offered better protection than either the "Morrison" or "Anderson" variety. There was also the added bonus that there was always the company of neighbours to share the danger.

If not playing board games with the other children, myself and Colleen used to make outline pictures on the floor with spent matches. Like most boys of my age I used to collect and swap shrapnel and one night, during a raid, I was standing as close to the shelter entrance as the adults would allow watching the searchlight beams in the sky and the flashes from either exploding ack ack shells or V1 impacts, when someone came into the shelter and presented me with a piece of shrapnel far larger than the usual pocket sized pieces the children usually collected. We assumed this was either because I was the lad closest to the entrance or that he was a friend of my parents. This piece bore one of the bars of the Swastika which was emblazoned on the tail fin of German aircraft, although I cannot now recall whether the line was a vertical or horizontal one. The possession of this made me the envy of other lads my age.

Other than when we had been transported between the various locations to which we were evacuated, Colleen and I saw no more of our father during the war than our compatriots whose fathers were in the services. My father was driving round the clock, seven days a week, from one end of the British Isles to the other.

The only recollection I have of wartime Christmases was probably in 1942 at which time I am sure we were located in Exeter. Late one night I can recall a tall figure entering the bedroom in which I shared a bed with my sister. The figure had snow on his shoulders and was carrying what appeared to be a gun. The next morning upon waking, at the end of the bed I discovered a wooden rifle in a pillow case together with an orange and a rag doll with a small wooden bed. Our father was home.

Like most of his contemporaries in the services my father, Len, did not say a great deal to his family of his experiences during the war years. However, some ten years or so after the war ended I found a bundle of letters that my mother had received from her husband during the war. I surreptitiously read their contents and became aware that what with the carnage caused on the roads as a result of having to drive without street lighting, coupled with the extremely long hours spent behind the wheel and the frequency with which either delivery or loading at the many ports and docks around the UK coincided with raids, my father's role in the conflict had been no easy one. The contribution he had made to the country's survival and final victory was by no means insignificant.

When the war in Europe came to an end in May 1945 the residents of Furley Road and the surrounding area prepared a large pyre of combustible material adjacent to the static water tank. In the evening a large crowd assembled to light the fire and watch the fireworks that had somehow been obtained for V.E. Day. It was during this evening that I sustained the only injury caused to any of the civilian members of the "Huzzey and Jago" clans. As part of the fireworks display a large Catherine Wheel had been vertically nailed to a plank and placed against the pyre prior to it being lit. When this was lit it spun around with increasing speed until it generated such force that it detached from the board, fell to the floor on its end and, still spinning, propelled itself across the ground until it met the toe of my shoe. It mounted the shoe and burnt a hole in my sock before I was yanked back out of harm's way.

In late 1945 or early 1946 my mother became pregnant with her third child, a boy, whom they named Terrance Leonard. The family moved back into 218 Cator Street, which had now been repaired from the blast damage sustained in 1940. We lived on the ground floor of the three-up, three-down, property with a childless couple, George and Peggy Elsey occupying the floor above. A second storey had been added to the downstairs scullery creating a kitchen/scullery at the upper level. The two families shared an outside toilet in the back yard. George was known to my father having at one point been his trailer mate. My father also claimed that, at one stage during the war, Frank Cousins, who later became General Secretary of the Transport & General Workers Union (TGWU), had also performed that role.

This return to Cator Street allowed Daisy's return to her parents' house from Exeter following her marriage. In early 1945 she had given birth to her and Bert's son Alan. Daisy was also desperate to return to London to be with

Bert who had been seriously injured during the battle for the liberation of Holland. He had been brought back to the U.K. where he needed an operation after being hit four times in the lower abdomen by bullets from a heavy machine gun. Much later I learned that Bert's operation had been performed by a German surgeon who had been taken prisoner in North Africa and was then working in Kings College Hospital in Camberwell, of which Peckham was a part. Five years later this hospital was to play a significant part in my own life.

After we have moved back to Cator Street it was found that, with the exception of my paternal grandparents at number 220, many of the neighbours from 1940 were no longer around. Next door, at number 216, lived a lady from Yorkshire together with her four sons and it was never clear whether she was widowed or separated. Her two eldest sons, Jack and Jim, had been in the navy, Bert, her third son had been in the army and then there was the youngest, Alan. In later years Alan's professional colleagues had referred to him as Alf taken from his initials. Alf Mason was around my age and the two of us became firm friends until we sadly lost contact with each other in the early 1980s.

We were both a constant source of puzzlement to the adult members of our respective families. Unlike our male contemporaries we were not interested in chasing a ball around, indulging in mock battles or games of tig, five stones, etc., but we would spend hours on the doorstep deep in earnest discussion on a whole range of subjects only ceasing once in a while to listen to the daily episode of either Dick Barton, Special Agent, or, Children's Hour if the current story being told was sufficiently absorbing to capture our interest. We were both avid readers and one of our first actions together was to join the public library. Alan soon became a keen Rider Haggard fan whilst I favoured W.E. Johns, author of the "Biggles" books.

Another activity we both enjoyed was exploring London on a Saturday within a radius we could comfortably manage. On one of our earlier expeditions we went missing for seven hours having made our way down through Bermondsey and across Tower Bridge to the north bank of the Thames. On the eastern shore, from the height of the road above the water, we saw what appeared to be a stretch of sand. Along the wharf, above the river, we eventually found the means to access this either via some steps or by means of a wide, heavily built ladder-like structure. When venturing forth onto what we assumed was sand we soon discovered that the sand was merely a light surface dusting over thick glutinous black mud. Alan, who had only been wearing sandals, suddenly lost his footing and sank up his thighs and although

I tried as hard as I could to try to pull him out I just couldn't. Shouting for help I clambered back up to the path and ran along the front of the wharf to seek adult assistance. Hearing my frantic cries two workers came out of the wharf and after looking in the direction in which I was pointing rushed back inside and quickly returned carrying a rope. Uncoiling the rope, at one end of which there was a small loop, the workers passed the other end of the rope through this loop thereby making a larger one. One of the men then climbed down the ladder and threw this loop towards Alan instructing him to pass it over his head and stretch his arms through. The man then instructed him to put his hands securely into his pockets and to make sure he kept them there. The man at the bottom then pulled the rope tight under Alan's shoulders and between them the two men pulled him out of the mud and hauled him up the ladder.

During the course of being dragged free of the clinging mud Alan lost one of his sandals so when he reached the path at the top, his rescuers bought a bucket of water and some rag and instructed him to wash himself off. While he was doing this the men asked where we had come from, how long we had been away from home and how we had gotten to the wharf. With our response the men told us there were no beaches on the Thames before Southend, there was only mud and, as Alan now knew to his cost, it was not suitable for paddling. We had both been very lucky; many other children, and indeed adults, had been sucked down under the mud. They warned us that we must never again attempt such an escapade.

Having by that time cleaned himself off Alan then had his sandal-less foot bound in rag with thick layers of cardboard tied to the base of his foot. We were then told to get the bus from the end of Tower Bridge back to Peckham. Upon learning that we had no money the men kindly gave us a shilling (5p) for bus fare. Passing on our sincere thanks to them for saving Alan we were sent on our way back home with strict instructions to remember what we had been told and to stick to dry land in future if we decided to go exploring again! When we got home we both "got it in the neck" from our mothers and Alan, in particular, from his two elder brothers. As former sailors they knew only too well how lucky he had been.

During the school holidays our explorations took us through the ruins around St Pauls which led to long discussions as to whether the cathedral's survival amidst such destruction was down to luck or divine intervention. We questioned the morality of mass bombing? As our discussions got deeper into the religious aspects, we began to wonder how much truth there was in the bible stories we were told at school. We both attended the Church of England school in Sumner Road which ran parallel to Cater Street. Our class teacher was a lady somewhat older and plumper than either of our mothers, who always seemed to wear a very heavy green dress.

Behind the school was a small park with a number of poplar trees, London Plane and a single conker tree. There were also a few houses, in front of which ran a path along the canal. One day I bought into school a conker case with the largest spikes I could find and placed it on the seat of the teacher's chair. The whole class watched in anticipation – would she see it? If not, would the spikes pierce the dress? With some disappointment the boys and girls watched as the teacher sat down seemingly quite unaware of anything unusual with her chair and proceeded to call their respective names for the daily class register.

Another piece of mischief that springs to mind is putting some "Reckits Blue" (a whitening agent or dye that our mothers used) into a small glass tube. Then, lying on the towpath under the canal bridge we would dip one hand into the water and flip a sickle back onto the path. We would then place it into the tube with a little water and replace the stopper. Two or three days later, with the stopper removed and the fish long dead, we would wave the tube under the noses of the girls in our class or hide it somewhere in the class-room where the putrid smell of decay would waft across the room.

From the small veranda-type balcony at the front of the bomb-blasted school in the middle section of Cator Street, together with a group of our classmates, we watched in fascination as wave after wave of aircraft flew over in the victory flypast. The children all enjoyed the spectacle, which was the only time in five years that anyone had enjoyed seeing so many planes flying over London without any fear. Most of the children found out later that their parents and relatives had not enjoyed it to quite the same degree.

At other times venturing down into the bottom end of Cater Street, I and two of my friends explored the shell of the damaged church. We found the main body of the church to be empty except at the end where what we assumed must have been the alter screen was leaning against the wall on the left hand side. Above the screen could be seen an open room and on climbing over the screen and entering the space above, in the far right hand corner we saw a ladder laid at an angle following the slope of the roof. At the end of this, in the dim light that filtered through displaced or broken slates, we could see a short vertical ladder leading into the belfry through which most of the light was coming. We proceeded to climb this ladder and, to our delight, found a single bell with its clapper still intact. The floor of the belfry was covered with dry pigeon droppings.

In the street below we could see a group of girls playing so we tolled the bell to gain their attention and then, when they looked in puzzlement towards the church, we gathered handfuls of the dried pigeon dung which we fashioned into balls and threw them down at the girls below. This game was repeated numerous times over the course of the school holidays. On the last occasion we attempted this bell ringing ruse to attract attention we received an unexpected surprise. From a nearby street, a policeman on a bike suddenly appeared heading for the church. Of course we all quickly descended to the base of the sloping ladder, dislodging enough tiles to enable us to gain access to the roof which had a gentle sloping angle at this point. We slid down the roof catching our heels in the guttering at the base, then jumped to the ground. The first two boys managed this successfully but, being taller and heavier, I hit my heels too hard into the gutter which promptly broke and without that support I fell to the ground.

As my friends made a run for it I dragged myself to my feet and with a tingling sensation in my arm decided that as Daisy's prefab was closer than home, I would go around to my aunt's. When I arrived there I found my uncle was also at home. I was asked why I was grimacing and on being told of the sensation in my arm was immediately questioned by Bert if I had fallen over. On examining my arm he got a wet tea towel which he wrapped round it. Later that evening, when I had returned home and the towel had been removed, my arm was found to be quite swollen so I was taken to the Accident and Emergency department of the local hospital where it was discovered that my arm was in fact fractured. This escapade bought about the end of the bomb site exploits.

Following this, to keep ourselves amused, Alan and I then settled down to museum visits with Hornimans in Dulwich soon whetting our appetites. We also became frequent visitors to the Science and Natural History Museum in Kensington. Additionally, a further and less dangerous haunt, if either of us had managed to save sufficient money – usually half a crown ($12^1/_2$p), was Foyles a second hand bookshop. We would easily spend a couple of hours in this shop diligently searching for books of interest often leaving with up to five books each. After reading them we would then swap with each other. This practice gave rise to more opportunities for further self education and discussion.

As the "11 plus" examinations approached the other children of our age were urged to concentrate on the main subjects. Sadly subjects like art, which was Alan's favourite, and woodwork/handicrafts, which was mine, were dropped. Sadly we had no option but to accept this but did so with mixed feelings. One of my woodworking achievements was to make a footstool which, although it had borne my own weight had unfortunately collapsed when my younger siblings decided they would join me on it.

For some years previous, under my father's instructions, it had been the practice for me to take my two younger siblings to Sunday School in the afternoon. Here each of us would be placed in a group with others of the same or similar age. Over the years I had developed the habit of using this as an opportunity to develop and enhance my debating skills. Whilst attending both a Church of England Junior School and also Sunday School, I was by no means convinced of the voracity of the stories and lessons the teachers in either establishment were seeking to put across. All the other children in my group would follow my challenges and question with interest the leader of the Sunday School class who faced this with despair. One Sunday evening when the family were sitting around the table eating our tea there was a knock on the front door. My father got up and went down the passage opening the door to a stranger whom he did not recognise. The man standing in front of him requested that he no longer send his eldest son to Sunday School and, when asked why, proceeded to give an explanation. My father then returned to the table and after relating to Nell, my mother, the essence of the conversation he had had on the doorstep turned to me and said, in effect, "if you think you are clever enough to challenge the teachers then make sure you pass the 11 plus!!"

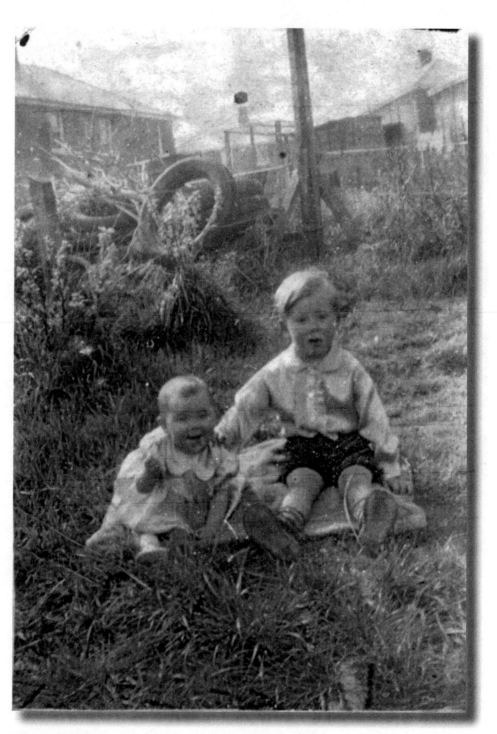

Me and Colleen (aged 8 months) in Exeter 1942

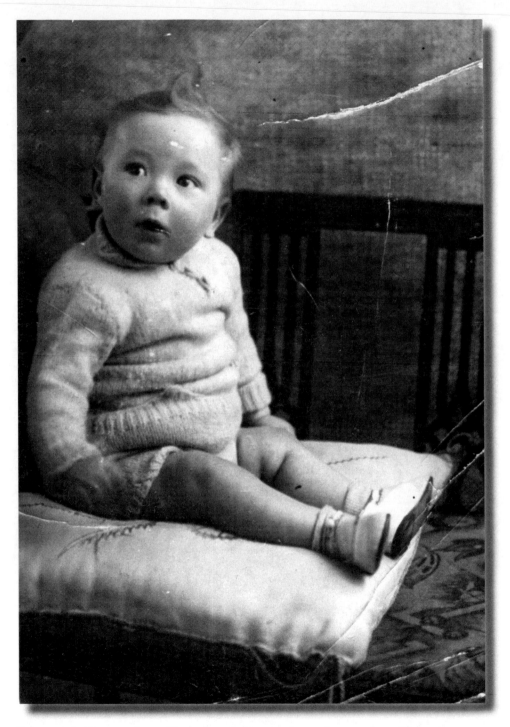

Me aged 15 months telling the photographer what to do – I've never changed!

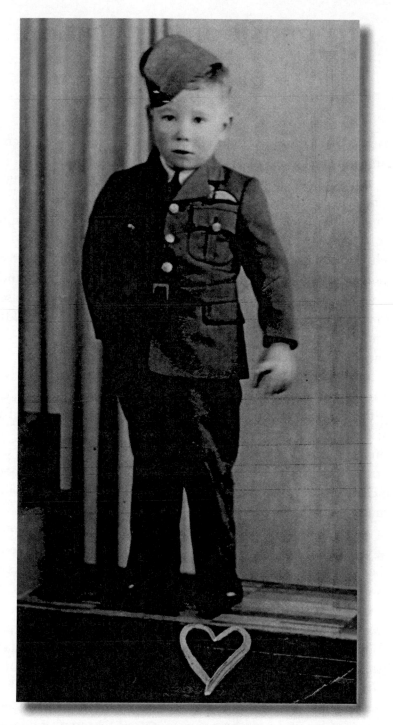

Me aged 5 pageboy at Bert and Daisy's wedding

Diagnosis and Education
in Diabetes

In early 1950 all the eldest pupils in the school sat the 11 plus examination. Alan came top in all of his subjects except for geography in which I beat him. He also attained equal grading with me in English. As a result, the grading system then in operation, meant that Alan passed for acceptance at grammar school with myself being borderline. Consequently Alan's mother was asked to accompany him for an interview at two local colleges in Aleynes and Dulwich. However she took exception to many of the questions asked of her in relation to her family background and as a consequence Alan found himself accompanying me into the grammar school stream at the local boys secondary modern school which was split over two sites, one for 12-13 year olds and the other for 14-15 year olds.

We now found ourselves in an all male educational environment and where we had previously shared a two person desk with a non-competitive girl we now found ourselves sitting next to boys who were, in some cases, extremely competitive. However, over the course of the July and August of that first year we both settled into this new environment reasonably well. Unfortunately in late August I started to become increasingly lethargic and was losing concentration. I was frequently on the receiving end of the wooden felt-backed chalk duster which the form master was in the habit of hurling across the room at any pupil he perceived not to be paying full attention.

One Saturday morning, around this time my mother asked me to take the bag containing the family's dirty clothing, sheets, etc., to the local bag wash, i.e. laundry (there was no such thing as washing machines available to the working class in 1950), drop it off and continue around to my nan's house then collect the clean wash on the way home. On arriving at my nan's I was greeted by the delicious and familiar aroma of rabbit stew. I petted and stroked "nigger", the dog, and exchanged greetings with my granddad and his old First World War comrade, Reg, who all remarked that I did not look too well. Nevertheless I was asked if I would like a dish of stew as that should "buck me up" and I agreed that I would like to try some. Later, when I left to collect the washing and head home, equal in today's terms of approximately the weight of three to four small bags of potatoes, I was feeling really awful. I could not see clearly and was guiding myself along by trailing my left hand along the brick walls of the house fronts. At every doorway I had to stop and reorient myself before being able to continue. I was also experiencing a raging thirst and stopping frequently to knock on doors to request a drink of water.

When I eventually arrived home, about ninety minutes after leaving my grandmother's, without the laundry and an hour later than expected, my mother was both alarmed and appalled at my appearance. I looked absolutely exhausted and had clearly wet myself a number of times. She immediately took me indoors, cleaned me up and put me straight to bed. She then hurried round to a telephone box and rang the doctor. Some time later the doctor had still not arrived and with me still calling for water, my father arrived home. He took one look at me and stormed out of the house angrily muttering that if necessary he would return dragging the doctor by the back of his neck.

The doctor duly arrived about ten minutes later having previously received my father's urgent demand. He knew from past experience gained over a long period as the family's G.P., that my father was not prone to exaggeration or someone to get on the wrong side of. Following his examination of me the doctor felt I was generally run down and should be kept in bed and given lemon and barley laced with plenty of sugar which, at that time, was still rationed. He undertook to call again in a few days' time to check on the patient.

I was then twelve years old, four feet, nine inches in height and weighing six stone. Four days later, with the house reeking of acetone and urine, no clean sheets or dry towels, and now weighing just twenty six pounds, I was deep in a ketotic coma. I was carried out of the house on a stretcher to a waiting ambulance. A neighbour two doors away, a mother of four, passed out at the sight of me and, some days later, said to my mother that I had looked like someone straight out of Belson.

Upon arrival at St Giles Hospital I was rushed into A&E where fortunately the duty doctor was Dr Philip Oakly, the Registrar to Dr Robin Lawrence the Consultant Endocrinologist at Kings College Hospital and the most eminent Diabetologist in Europe. Dr Oakly knew immediately what was wrong with me but thought the case sufficiently urgent to call in Dr Lawrence. I was subsequently told by my parents what had transpired. A limousine screamed to a halt at the entrance to the A&E department and an imposing figure dressed in a black suite and tails hurried inside and went straight through to the surgery. He emerged about an hour later to inform them that their son had insulin dependent diabetes and was gravely ill. He promised he would do all in his power to succeed in stabilising my condition but my chances of living beyond another thirty six hours were not high.

I have recently received the Lawrence Medal awarded to people who have survived for sixty years with Type One diabetes. This story is an account of what that great doctor achieved and the knowledge and confidence he instilled into me to enable me to go on to great achievements in my life.

To give an indication of the scale of this, statistically there are in the order of 125,000 Type One diabetics in the U.K. at any one time. I believe this equates to 7.5 million people who have been diagnosed with the condition since 1950. I am the 399th person to have received this medal, therefore the odds are 188,000 to one against. The purpose of this story is to pass on to those newly diagnosed with this condition, particularly youngsters, the most important lesson of **"strict carbohydrate control"**!

I remained in hospital for a period of six weeks. On regaining consciousness, thirty six hours after admission, I felt pressure on my hand and heard a soft voice which I did not recognise. I distinctly recall this voice saying "welcome back Tony". I was asked to open my eyes and I saw a young girl in a white hat and dress sitting by my bedside. I could not move my legs and when I was lifted up with pillows placed behind me to prop me up, at the end of the bed I saw a long glass tube the end of which was in my ankle. Now, after sixty years, the scar this left has completely vanished and I am not sure now whether it was on the left or right ankle. My legs had been strapped to the bed and I was receiving nutriments, i.e. insulin and glucose, via this source direct into my bloodstream.

My parents were frequently at my bedside and were finally told their son was out of danger but needed to sleep to give my body time to regain all the body tissue it had lost. My body had ceased to produce insulin which was needed to convert food to energy. This energy would normally be supplied by the food group called "carbohydrates" like bread, cereals, root vegetables, fruit, etc., which, when utilised by insulin gave the body the power it needed. In the absence of that insulin my body needed an alternative fuel source in order for me to keep breathing and for my heart to keep beating. I had burnt off all my body fat and most of my muscle tissue. This had produced both the acetone stench and my skeletal appearance. I would need at least a couple of weeks of intense nutritional treatment via the drip to regain my former appearance. However my parents would see improvements in my condition on a daily basis whilst undergoing this treatment.

My parents were obviously very distraught at this whole situation and both had tears in their eyes as they tried to absorb this information. They were assured that I would be allowed to eat as soon as I was able to but henceforth would be on a strictly controlled diet and would need insulin injections every day for the rest of my life.

Over the course of my stay in hospital I became great friends with this nurse who was known as "Bridey O'Toole". Type One diabetes had entered my life at exactly the medium age range that the condition usually manifested itself at that time.

For the next four or five days, as I lay in bed, I recalled in my imagination the great excitement of my twelfth birthday. Mum had insisted that I had my photograph taken in my school uniform and after much protesting I finally conceded to her request on the proviso that Prince could also be in the picture since it must also coincide with his tenth birthday.

We had been staying in a boarding house in Ramsgate and my father, as he usually did, turned first to the back page of his Herald, leaving the news until he had perused the runners and riders at the day's horse or dog race meetings. Sitting opposite to him I was therefore able to see the headlines on the front page. These proclaimed that the Americans had landed in Korea. With my interest in geography I knew that it was some 6,000 miles from the coast of the U.S.A. I asked my father what right they had to do this. Why were they interfering? Was it not up to the Koreans to sort out their own affairs? The two other families in the boarding house listened in some surprise as an animated discussion developed on this subject between father and son across the dining room.

We had been eating breakfast when my father asked me what I wanted for my birthday. Each morning after we had arrived at the boarding house I had watched fascinated as a small Auster single engine plane had flown low over the beach and harbour heading west along the coast then turning over the sea towards the Dogger Bank and returning via Margate to Manston Airfield. I had seen these flights advertised on bill boards together with pleasure boat or fishing trips. I responded that I would very much like to take that flight. My mother was horrified and my father was somewhat reluctant to agree. Neither one had ever flown, nor did they ever fly during their lifetime. However my father persuaded my mother to agree to my request pointing out to her that Charlie, his younger brother who was a Lancaster pilot during the war, had always told him that his first ever flight in a Tiger Moth during his training in Canada had been one of the greatest experiences of his life. Lying there in bed with my eyes firmly closed I re-lived that fifteen minute flight over and over again.

Dad paid the equivalent of, in today's money, £2.50 for this flight. I was taken from the office to the plane where I had to climb a pair of steps as tall as myself and go through a small door onto a seat alongside the pilot. Strapping me in he introduced himself as Ken and asked what my name was. He told me to relax, turned a key and after a couple of coughs the propeller began to spin gradually getting faster and faster. Then, with Ken explaining what would happen the plane began to move forward across the field. Just as I thought we would hit the rapidly approaching hedge Ken pulled back the lever between his knees and, to my great surprise, we rose over the hedge at the field boundary. Looking to my left I suddenly realised we were airborne.

As the Auster climbed I was enthralled to find myself looking down on a farmhouse where the cows in the yard seemed to be no bigger than ants. As we approached Ramsgate the layout of the streets and houses brought to mind the pictures that Colleen and I had made with matchsticks when we had taken refuge in the shelter during the war years. We then flew lower over the beach and I could see the people sitting under the pavilion to avoid sunburn and the children playing and digging in the sand. The open air lido at the end of the beach was fascinating because I could see people swimming under the water just like the grey mullet in the waters of the inner harbour at the opposite end of the beach. At the water's edge I could see the waves travelling from far offshore and follow them as they rolled in to finally crash onto the beach where they swept forward to where the children laughingly jumped over them. I watched fascinated as one beach ball was carried out far beyond the harbour entrance. As Ken turned the plane I looked down onto the rocky shore where I spent most mornings searching rock pools for hermit crabs, whelks and sea urchins to take back in a bucket to show my little brother Len who was then only five years old and not allowed to accompany me on my lone excursions.

As we approached Pegwell Bay to fly over the Viking longboat on its stand above the beach, I proudly told Ken that I had watched as it had come in two years earlier. Turning left, Ken then headed the plane out into the channel, climbing until I could clearly see to the left the sandbanks of the Goodwins and the French coast to the right. As we banked again and headed back to Manston I asked Ken how high we had flown and he responded with three hundred feet. Although I was later to work on buildings much higher, sixty years on I fondly remember the thrill of that flight which was the first time I had ever been so high.

After some days, now becoming more wakeful, I awoke to find a number of doctors around my bed. The eldest amongst them was explaining to the others the background to my current situation. Realising I was awake and listening to the conversation this doctor indicated for the others to continue with the ward round whilst he remained to speak with the patient alone. He introduced himself to me as Dr Robin Lawrence and continued by saying he knew how I must be feeling and what I had gone through as he had gone through the same thing himself some thirty years ago when he was just a young doctor. He said that like him, I would learn to live with and manage the condition because he was going to teach me how to do so providing I was willing to learn. He said this with a stern look on his face but always maintaining eye contact with me. In my customary challenging manner, I asked him what would happen if I was not willing to learn. He looked at Bridie O'Toole, who had joined him at my bedside, then turned his gaze back to me saying "you are twelve aren't you, but if you are not prepared to learn then you will not see your thirteenth birthday." This straightforward, no nonsense approach, established a deep and long lasting respect between us that was maintained for the next ten years.

As I have now realised many years later, amongst his varied skills, Dr Lawrence was no mean judge of childhood psychology, and had placed me in the men's, rather than the children's, ward at St Giles. He asked me how I felt about injections and I responded that I wanted to see my thirteenth birthday. Dr Lawrence was pleased with my response because he told me that I would have to inject myself twice a day, every day, for the rest of my life.

Turning to Bridie, Dr Lawrence asked her to bring him the hose and syringe as he wanted to give me my first lesson. Bridie returned carrying half a meter of red rubber tubing, a glass syringe 1.5 centimetres in diameter, a needle about the size and length of a darning needle, a small glass tube with a rubber cap and a small gritstone. Dr Lawrence checked each item in turn and told me I could practice using them until the following evening. By then, if I was able to inject myself, he would remove the tube from my ankle. Bridie was going to show me how to do it and Dr Lawrence told me he had every confidence that I would succeed. He then left my bedside and went off to join the other doctors on the ward round.

Bridie proceeded to show me the barrel of the syringe, the body of which contained a series of short black lines. She explained that each line represented two units and that I needed to depress the plunger to correspond to the requisite number of units I had to take. It was important that I inspected the liquid in the syringe to make sure there was no air bubble present. It there was then I would have to push the plunger down until the bubble disappeared then draw down again to the number of units I had to take. I had to repeat this procedure until I was absolutely certain that everything was OK and it was safe to proceed. This was a vitally important rule which must always be followed to the letter. Even the most experienced doctors and nurses sometimes hit a blood vessel when injecting patients and the consequences would be very dangerous if an air bubble was inadvertently injected into the blood stream.

Bridie also showed me how to use the small gritstone to sharpen the needle which, after being used for a number of times, would lose its sharp point and develop a barbed end making it difficult to insert and very painful to pull out.

When my mother came to see me that evening she told me that my father had been unable to come with her as he couldn't get back in time from his day's trip. I later discovered, however, that he had in fact been pulled over for speeding. She looked on with something approaching horror on her face and showed great concern when she realised that I was practising with the rubber tube the injection process I would, the following evening, have to do on myself. Even at that young age I was fully aware that my mother had enough on her plate with looking after my father, brother Len, and sister Colleen, without this added worry. At that point I became fully resolved to take responsibility of managing my diabetes myself. I was determined to follow Dr Lawrence's example and not let this condition beat me. I would learn all I could about it and whilst I could obviously not stop my parents from worrying, which was only natural, I could at least alleviate the pressures on them by taking control of my own treatment. As the eldest of the three children I felt it was my duty to set them a good example by showing them that we all have to live up to the responsibilities of our own lives.

The following evening Bridie brought with my dinner, a syringe and vial of insulin and drew the curtains around my bed. She told me how much insulin I needed to inject and checked my legs to make sure I had sufficient flesh on my thighs in which to insert the needle. She then demonstrated how I should squeeze a piece of flesh between the finger and thumb of my left hand whilst, with my right hand, insert the needle at a forty five degree angle which was necessary in order to facilitate the length of the needle. Following her guidance I completed the task and a pleased Bridie opened the curtains saying in a voice far louder than previously "there, you have done it"! To my amazement there then followed a round of applause from the other patients on the ward who were capable of clapping their hands and shouts of "well done" from those who could not.

Dr Lawrence's clever tactic of placing me on the men's ward soon paid immediate dividends as my confidence soared under the praise and encouragement I received from the adult patients. When my parents came to see me later during visiting hours, telling them of my success, their relief was clearly evident and they went home that evening feeling much happier than at any time over the last three weeks and optimistic that their son's future would possibly be brighter than they had previously feared.

The next morning, after successfully injecting myself for a second time, Dr Lawrence inspected the areas of my self-injection attempts and congratulated me on not producing any bruising. He also advised me on the most appropriate areas of my body for injection, i.e. thighs, biceps, buttocks and waist, and stressed the importance of alternating my injections around all of these areas. The drip in my ankle was then removed and a dressing applied. That done, my next lesson on diabetes was delivered.

I needed to understand that the bodies of people with diabetes took longer to heal from wounds and any that were sustained had to be checked frequently to make sure they did not become septic which could result if blood sugar levels were not kept under control. In 1950 the method used to determine blood sugar levels was to test a urine sample. This procedure had to be learnt and practised over the course of the next nine weeks.

Having been in bed since I had, with so much difficulty, walked home from my grandmother's house, I asked if I could finally get up. Whilst no longer skeletal, I was still a long way from regaining the weight of a normal twelve year old but I was given permission to try. Dr Lawrence warned me not to expect too much at this stage and positioned himself at the head of my bed. Bridie then proceeded to swing my legs off the bed. Placing my feet on the floor I was told to try to stand up and walk to her where she was standing at the foot of my bed. Placing my hands on the edge of the bed and using my arms for support I pushed myself upright and turned to face Bridie who was waiting anxiously at the end of the bed. I slowly lifted my foot to take a step forward and promptly fell straight into her outstretched arms. This came as no surprise to either of the medics and I was gently advised not to despair but to return to bed and arrangements would be made for a physiotherapy nurse to come and give me some exercises to strengthen my muscles and when I was strong enough I could try again.

Many of the men on my ward were former servicemen who had been injured in combat. They assured me that exercise would enable me to regain the ability to walk and run. More than a few also expressed their admiration at my ability to self inject which was something they could or would not be able to do.

With this encouragement and a lot of hard work, within a week I was walking round the ward. I had also learnt how to play whist and solo which are still my card games of choice today. When not playing cards I could usually be found in the ward kitchen using the flexible gas stove lighting torch to singe the cockroaches crawling up the walls in there. If I was not playing cards or frying cockroaches I usually ensconced myself in reading "Thor Heyerdahl's Kon Tiki Expidition", a paperback edition of which my Uncle Charles had persuaded one of his Trans Atlantic pilot colleagues to pick up in New York. My Uncle was then flying the European routes and arranged to get me this book after I had asked my father if he could get it for me from the library. I had become interested in the Kon Tiki expedition from listening to the radio through the headphones from my hospital bed.

On the outside of the ward there was an iron fire escape running down to the ground from a small balcony/platform. The hospital stood inside a ten feet high wall which isolated it from the surrounding streets. One evening I asked my parents if they could arrange for Len and Colleen to stand on the street corner, which could be seen from the balcony. So, to our joint delight, my brother and sister, together with my best friend, duly appeared on that street corner. Sadly the distance was too great for conversation but we managed to confirm that we were all OK and with shouts and waves conveyed our joy and happiness at seeing each other again after five long weeks.

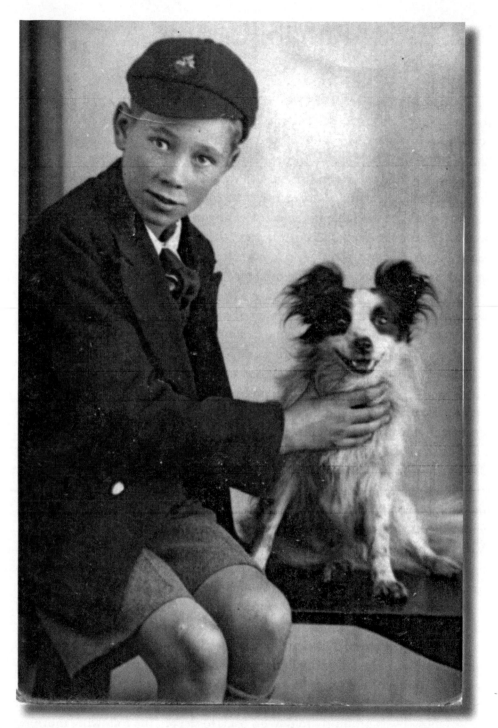

Me on my 12th Birthday with Prince 8 weeks before diabetes struck

Rehabilitation

In order to start my formal education into diabetes control and mastering the techniques and practises I needed to learn to enable me to live with the condition, it was recommended to my parents that I spend three weeks at a home/school in Birchington on the Kent coast. There, together with up to twelve other children around my age, I would be given the knowledge and the supervised opportunity to practise these methods where qualified medical support would be available in the event of any problems arising. All the children were accommodated in dormitories at this home and had access to the beach for exercise and play. My parents were assured, however, that not until we had become more proficient would we have access to the sea.

So it was that six weeks after being admitted to St Giles close to death I found myself saying an emotional farewell to Bridie and thanking all the men on my ward who had given me so much support and encouragement, in addition to teaching me to play the card game of solo! There was however yet one further experience which would impress upon me the importance of understanding and mastering the art of living with Type One diabetes. Some two weeks prior to my leaving the hospital a twenty year old man named Brian was brought in unconscious and placed in the bed next to mine around which the curtains were drawn closed. Bridie told me later that he had the same condition as myself but did not follow the rules. The next day, following his return to consciousness, I heard him being scolded by the doctors. When I talked to him later on he told me that he resented the fact he had this condition and was determined to follow the same lifestyle he had enjoyed before his diagnosis. When my parents came to see me that evening my father greeted him and told me later that Brian was the son of one of the men who used the same pub as him. Apparently Brian "liked a pint" which was the root cause of his problem.

Brian had been admitted to the ward late on a Friday night and discharged the following Monday morning having received another scolding from the doctors who had urged him that he must change his ways if he wanted to continue to live. The following Friday night I was woken up around midnight by the slamming of the ward doors. I was aware of light shining from torches and of the curtains being opened around the next bed. On catching sight of me watching I was promptly told to go back to sleep. The following morning Bridie made a point of coming to tell me that Brian had again been admitted but that would be his last admission; despite the huge efforts of the night staff they had been unable to save him and Brian had died during the early hours of the morning. This was to prove a salutary lesson for me.

My father had borrowed a car for the journey to Birchington and for the first time in six weeks, for a couple of hours at least, we were again a reunited family of five. We all made the most of this precious time together and chatted happily during the car ride which was a unique experience in itself for my mother and both my siblings.

Upon arrival we found the home at Birchington to be a large three-storey detached house located away from other smaller houses on the seafront. We entered through one of the two large double doors at the entrance and stepped into a room with a brown tiled floor and a wide staircase on the right hand side of the entrance. This led to a landing from the left hand side of which the staircase continued on to a higher floor above. The smell of boiled cabbaged mixed with something else greeted us and both Colleen, and Len in particular, screwed up their noses in disgust which was a facial habit all three of us had inherited from our father. Somewhat shocked, mother had identified the other smell and turning to father whispered that it was "piss"! A rather plump lady wearing a black dress with a shawl-like white collar and a wide white belt around her waist entered the rather gloomy room from a door on our left. She introduced herself as the matron and asked my father for my name. She then invited us all to follow her into her office. She pointed to a padded light green seat in the large bay window and in a soft voice told Colleen to sit there. Turning to Len, who was then nearly five years old, she told him more sternly to "sit, not stand". This was said however with a smile and reaching into a desk drawer she retrieved a comic which she handed to Colleen and a picture book which she passed to Len. She then asked my parents and myself to sit on the seats in front of her desk, sitting herself behind it.

Turning to me she then said "I am told that you do your own injections" to which I nodded yes. She picked up a piece of paper and told my parents that Dr Lawrence had written to her advising that I would be a good example to, and a great help in supporting the other children. She then asked me if it was correct that I had already been practising urine testing to which I again nodded my assent. I was surprised to see my father's face flush with what he later told me was pride, whilst my mother brushed away a tear with her cuff.

We were then shown to the room that I would be staying in for the duration of my stay where mother unpacked my clothes either hanging them in the wardrobe or laying them neatly in the drawers. She instructed me how to use them stressing that I must always ensure I wore clean vests and pants.

Sadly the time eventually came for my family to leave and I can remember tearfully waving them goodbye from the staircase landing. Equally tearful they left by the front door with promises to return in about three weeks' time or sooner if possible.

At this point in my narrative I must make note of a sudden awareness that has just occurred to me sixty years later. From recalling the events in my life that I am describing here I have realised how deeply impressed upon my subconscious mind they are, particularly the waking awareness and sight of that special lady, Bridie O'Toole. Those of you who are reading, and I hope enjoying, my attempt to record my autobiography, will appreciate the meaning of this point if, as I hope you will, stay with me to the end of my book.

The group of children, of which I was one, who were staying at the home at the time, numbered around ten or twelve and we all came from a variety of different places across the south of the country. Aged between eleven and thirteen years old, all of us had arrived within days of each other. The first time we assembled together was before breakfast the day after my arrival when we were all asked to stand in line and role up the sleeve of our pyjamas so that we could be given our respective injections. As I already knew how to self inject, and indeed had been doing so for the past two weeks, I objected, protesting that I would administer my own injection. This fiercely independent stance was one I would frequently adopt throughout my life when I found myself challenged with what I felt was an unnecessary instruction.

Much to my surprise I was told that the other children had not yet been similarly taught. I was asked by the nurse if I was also able to draw up the correct quantity of insulin I needed to inject and when I answered in the affirmative she handed me the syringe and vial of insulin. She told me the number of units required and summoned the others to watch. Needless to say they all watched in fascination as I placed the needle in the vial, expelled the air and drew down the syringe plunger to the ninth mark for eighteen units. As I had been taught I checked the syringe for any air bubbles, pushed the plunger down to the eighth mark, pinched up the flesh on my thigh and, with an audible "wow" from my captivated audience, I duly administered my own injection. With a smile I then turned and handed the syringe back to the nurse. With that she said to the other children, "there, you are all the same age and all need to inject; if Tony can do it you can too. Today he will help me to teach you how, won't you Tony"? She gave me a smile of encouragement as I nodded in agreement.

Following this we all proceeded to go in for breakfast which consisted of a bowl of thick porridge. The matron joined us and asked me how I had learned to self inject to which I duly responded. After breakfast she returned with short lengths of tube, a box of needles and enough syringes for everyone to have one each. Together with the nurse I spent the rest of that first day helping her teach the other children how to inject themselves. After lunch, with the use of a bowl of water, the afternoon was spent practising the procedure of expelling air and drawing off a measured dose. That evening those who felt confident enough were allowed to inject themselves with the ones who felt less confident continuing to practise as before until it was time for bed. I now realise this was, in essence, a practical example of what was to become the firm political, economic and moral philosophy of my life. From each according to his ability; to each according to his need!

Whilst this may sound pretentious to the reader, I had been fortunate enough to have been taught to be self reliant insofar as injections were concerned, my colleagues had not. I had been invited to assist them to gain the necessary skill and confidence and was only too happy to comply. We were all in the same boat and, henceforth, this was something we would all have to do every day for the rest of our lives.

The next morning we were each handed our own syringe, needle and vial of insulin and told how much we needed to inject. Under the scrutiny of the nurse and the matron we all did as we had been instructed. Following successful completion of the task we all happily congratulated each other and then with much happy laughter and very few tears we ate our porridge in readiness for our next important lesson.

In the 1950's, unlike today, one had to determine the amount of sugar in one's body by measuring the quantity contained in a urine sample. This involved placing a sample of urine into a test tube which was then mixed with a blue liquid called Benidict Solution. The test tube then had to be heated by either holding it over a bunsen burner or immersing it into boiling water (this elicited the smell that caused our noses to wrinkle) until the mixture changed colour. If it remained blue then no sugar was present and if that was the case then one needed to eat something containing carbohydrates. If an injection was due when the test was done then a meal had to be eaten first before the injection was administered which was the reverse of the usual procedure. If the mixture in the test tube turned green that meant there was a trace of sugar, if it turned orange this indicated that the levels were too high and if it turned brown then this meant there were excessive, and potentially dangerous, levels of sugar in your system.

Now that we had all achieved the same level of training our first week was spent learning this skill and the value of carbohydrate foods, identifying which ones contained carbohydrates and which ones contained fats and proteins.

Prior to this however we were all allowed to go to the beach to enjoy a game of rounders or cricket accompanied by the matron and the nurse who were armed with barley sugar sweets. This was a necessary precaution in case anyone, being released from the confines of the home and associated lessons, became too over-boisterous resulting in an insulin reaction that was known at that time as a hyperglycaemic attack (or hypo in short).

On that sunny mid September afternoon, with a firm shingle beach crunching under our feet and a cooling refreshing breeze blowing off the sea, we all made the most of the welcome release from the confines of the various hospital wards we had been cooped up in over the past few weeks; coming together from different hospitals located in different parts of the country. We all cried out in delight, shouting and laughing with some of us attempting handstands, some kicking up the sand in sheer joy and others making a beeline for the water's edge. Many of these children were visiting the beach for the first time and it was a completely new experience for them. On examining the dry weed and detritus gathered at the high tide mark these children cried out in alarm when sand hoppers and the occasional crab scuttled out of the sea. They were also unfamiliar with the angry seagulls that swooped down at those of us who were disturbing what they regarded as their property. A little way off from our group a couple of people exercising their dogs on leads looked on in perplexity at this group of noisy children who were seemingly running riot on the normally quiet beach.

A whistle suddenly rang out and with the school discipline instilled in each of us we stopped and turned to where the nurse was waving and beckoning us to her side. When we all gathered around her the matron proceeded to check her list of the urine test samples we had each recorded. Most of us, but not all, had results showing either blue or green and were duly handed a barley sugar with the strict instruction to suck it slowly and make it last and on no account were we to bite or swallow it. Then, so that both the matron and the nurse could keep us all in their sights, we had to split ourselves into two teams for a game of rounders. Those not having received a barley sugar were to do all the running. Thus we learned by practical example how exercise can lower the blood sugar. At the end of the afternoon we returned to the home where we performed the required urine test and when matron had recorded all the results were told how much insulin we each needed to inject.

In our third and final week at Birchington we were to receive instruction on the different types of food, i.e. carbohydrate, protein and fats, and an introduction to a system of dietary control of our condition that had been devised by Dr Lawrence who, having the condition himself since 1922, had perfected it by experimenting on himself.

This system was based on five gram quantities of each different food types. From our point of view, as Type One diabetics, carbohydrates were the most important to understand since the body immediately converted them to glucose and it was the glucose level in the body that we needed to control by way of the injection. Since the capacity of our bodies to produce our own insulin had been destroyed, we had to learn to live our lives by keeping things in balance. Too much of any one of these three food types, or indeed too little, would cause us problems and it was these three "demons" that we needed to control : carbohydrates - eaten; insulin – injected; exercise – taken.

Given the average twelve year old normally has a healthy appetite, and I was no exception, I will give a couple of examples of alternative foods containing five grams of carbohydrate, i.e. one third of an ounce of bread, three ounces of raw carrot, one ounce of potato, six ounces of swede (boiled) or, if really hungry, 17.5 ounces of boiled cabbage.

In 1950 food was still subject to wartime rationing and by no means as plentiful as we enjoy today. There were no supermarkets back then and very little choice or variety. However, as children, there was one thing we all had in common, diabetic or not, at the end of a meal we all had clean plates!

We also learned how an adverse reaction (hypo) felt. This was usually experienced by profuse sweating, irrespective of ambient temperature, the loss of controlling movement to our arms and legs or, in extreme circumstances, the confusion and inability to think clearly and the drowsiness preceding a lapse into unconsciousness. These last two symptoms also manifested when hyperglycaemia (too high a sugar level) was threatening. I have always regarded the second of these as by far the worst, robbing me of the ability to function at all whereas I find I can function reasonably well all through "hypo" (by scientific definition).

During the early afternoon of the Friday of that third week my family returned to Birchington to take me home. When they arrived we all happily hugged each other in turn, not without a few tears but also with many happy smiles. Matron duly informed my parents that true to Dr Lawrence's report about me in his letter to her, I had indeed set an example to the other children who, with the encouragement they needed, all demonstrated their eagerness to follow and learn from my example. She told them that she would, in turn, respond to Dr Lawrence in writing giving him a full report of my success at which I saw my father's face really light up.

Sadly, following my goodbyes to all those other children with whom I had shared the past three weeks, I have never seen any of them again. However I did hear, some time later, that two of them had also married at around the same time as myself. Consequently I would request that if anyone reading this has any relations or friends who were at the Birchington Convalescent Home for diabetic children in September 1950 then I would very much appreciate their getting in touch,

With the good wishes of the matron and staff echoing in my ears I gladly climbed into the back seat of what I believe was a black Standard Vanguard that my father had borrowed to come and collect me. So, with unending questions from my brother and sister, we headed for home from which I had been absent for the past nine weeks.

Upon presenting ourselves at the heavy green front door and whilst my mother was searching in her purse for the key, all I could hear was excited barking and frantic scratching coming from inside. As mother pushed fruit-lessly at the door my father stepped forward and yelled through the letterbox for Prince to get away and with a mighty thump of his hand pushed the door open. At this a sudden flash of black and white shot through the opening between my father's feet and leapt into my outstretched arms. Following my father indoors I was surprised how much lighter the normally dark passage appeared from what I remembered. This impression of light was the first of several significant changes that had occurred within the house during my nine weeks of absence of which no-one had breathed a word to me on our journey home.

Adjusting to Life With Diabetes

Opening the second door on the left and entering the room I was again surprised to find there was no bed in there and seeing my startled expression my mother said "first things first, your father and I need a cup of tea, how about you?". Over a welcome cup of tea I was told that the couple who had previously lived upstairs (Peggy and George) had now moved out following very forcible representations my mother had made to the Housing Authority. She had stressed that her three children, including a girl of ten and boys aged twelve and five, were crammed into the constraints of the four rooms which our family occupied. This imposed on them the necessity of three children having to share the same bedroom. Additionally there was now the added problem that their eldest had been diagnosed with diabetes and her daughter must have a room of her own. The Housing Authority had agreed, hence the removal of Peggy and George. Consequently Colleen now occupied what was their former bedroom leaving myself and my brother Lennie to occupy what had previously been their kitchen/dining room.

As my mother had accompanied the family to collect me from the home she had not had an opportunity to prepare any dinner. So as this was a special day with us all being reunited it was decided we would celebrate with what, for the past five years, had been regarded as a rare treat – fish and chips. This did not require the use of ration coupons but was also not controlled by fixed prices so therefore could not often be afforded by the ordinary working class family.

Mother had instructed Colleen to apply some surgical spirit to a wad of cotton wool on the spot on my body I had decided to do my injection but looked away as I carried out the procedure. This was the start of my family's involvement in my condition and during those first weeks back home I was frequently asked if I had either tested my urine or administered my injection. Things soon settled down however and these questions were only raised when and if my behaviour started to seem a little odd or out of character.

The following morning after my first day home my urine level tested orange; I had not yet developed the knowledge which would allow me to look at a pile of chips for example and make an accurate estimation of the two ounce portion I could safely devour. I had also not taken into account the batter that encased the fish. Therefore, with the little skill I had already attained I injected my usual amount of insulin, ate a smaller breakfast than usual and told my mother I was going out to take a walk around the block. By lunch time my urine level showed green.

My mother had received a letter from Kings College Hospital inviting us to attend the diabetic clinic so she sensibly suggested I should write down my test colours to take along with us. On my first morning at home we duly attended the clinic and after walking along a series of corridors for some ten minutes with our nostrils picking up the same smell we had noticed upon our arrival at Birchington, we eventually turned right into another corridor, handed in our invitation letter and were invited to take a seat in the waiting area. We slowly moved along the row of seating, taking the ones next to ours as they become vacant, heading towards a large room at the bottom. Once we entered this room we would have to wait until my name was called, approximately about an hour. Firstly though I had to be weighed and provide a urine sample. The result of the weighing went some way to reassuring my mother for whilst I had not completely regained my pre-diagnoses weight I was not too far off this.

When we eventually entered the large room we saw over one hundred people waiting, very few of whom were children. At the front of the room was a large piece of apparatus from which originated the smell that had permeated our nostrils when we arrived, i.e. the Benedict solution and urine. On entry to the room a blood sample was taken from me which would determine a more accurate level of my glucose (sugar) level than the urine test. Much earlier than we expected, my name was called and my mother and I were ushered through to a desk behind which sat Dr Philip Oakley. The first words he directed at my mother were "he looks much better than he did when I last saw him". With a grateful smile on her face she happily agreed. He went on to tell us that before we left we would be informed how much carbohydrate I should eat each day, broken down into amounts per meal and also how much short and long acting insulin I should inject and when. He then told us that after we had seen Dr Lawrence the Almoner would give my mother the following items:-

- a set of small scales.
- a stainless steel template to be used for measuring the amount of bread I was allowed to eat,
- sheets of paper showing the weight of various foods I could eat to correspond with the diet Dr Lawrence would set for me.

Dr Oakley said I would be seen on a monthly basis until the New Year when hopefully there would perhaps not be the need for such frequent visits to the clinic.

When we finally saw Dr Lawrence he told my mother that he had just received a telephone call from the matron at the home in Birchington who had confirmed that I had indeed lived up to his expectations. He also told her that she should not worry unduly about her son who understood the serious nature of his condition and showed a keenness to learn all he could about it. He reassured her that I was going to manage O.K.

The daily carbohydrate intake I was then given would be two hundred grams with sixteen units of soluble insulin and four units of protamine zinc insulin of eighty units per cc strength, both morning and evening. Dr Lawrence handed me a 10cc vial of the two types and instructed me to draw up the soluble first then the 4PZ1 making sure not to expel the soluble into the PZ1 vial. A ratio of one unit of insulin per five grams of carbohydrate. I have broadly followed this ratio for the past sixty years and am pleased to report that I have retained my sight and can still walk at least a mile, albeit with great difficulty. Whilst I have experienced two minor strokes and one cardiac arrest, following the rules and advice I received as a twelve year old has allowed me to do this. Any parent reading this should consider demanding their child be given the same opportunity.

In the early post war years a tradition had been established which continued into the late 1950s. The evening/night of Christmas Day would be spent at our maternal grandmother's house with the extended family of the Jago clan meeting for a "boozy" evening's entertainment of singing, dancing and general home made fun. These occasions invariably ended very late when my father and two of my mother's cousins-in-law would, with a burnt cork, decorate the face of our grandfather who, after a couple of drinks, always fell asleep in an armchair. This was carried out under the direction of Reg, my grandfather's wartime comrade from the trenches in the 1914-18 war. On being nudged awake and with a mirror being dangled in front of his face, he would mutter and swear at his son-in-law something along the lines of "bloody Huzzey", then burst out laughing with the comment "Reg, they've done it again!".

Boxing night was spent with the extended Huzzey clan at the home of our Uncle Charlie. This gathering would usually be quieter than the one on the previous night, the evening being spent playing family games, charades, etc. On both of these festive occasions I would be the eldest of the children that were present. Christmas 1950 was destined to be my biggest challenge since being diagnosed with diabetes. My immediate family understood my rejection of almost all the usual Christmas treats on offer but, on that first Christmas as a diabetic, my uncles, aunts and cousins were perplexed. By 1951, with many of the wartime restrictions now lifted and one year's diabetic experience behind me, I would accept the occasional tangerine, brazil or walnut.

However another problem presented itself. Many of our various aunts had made the effort to seek out so-called diabetic products and I soon became the recipient of numerous bars of chocolate and jars of marmalade and jam so labelled. It is now argued that these products are unnecessary and provided those with Type One diabetes, who may be reading this, use normal jams / marmalades only exceedingly frugally and take a walk after doing so to help the body absorb the sugar content, then I would support this practice.

However, diabetic chocolate in those days presented a different proposition. It was dark and hard with no trace of sweetness whatsoever with only the taste of its cocoa bean source. My siblings and cousins, aunts and uncles, mother and father, tasted it only once and all pulled grimacing faces and asked me in disgust and disbelief how I could eat it. My response would be a shrug of my shoulders with a reply of "not very often" or "sparingly".

Bearing this in mind, Christmas has always proved a difficult time since even the most resolute of us, at some time or another, will err. I was no exception. So, depending upon my test results I would either have to increase my insulin dose, reduce my carbohydrate intake or go for a long walk. Frequently, as the years have passed, and I have subsequently become a father myself, I have found that a combination of all three has become necessary. This was especially the case on Boxing Day mornings when I would be left with no alternative but to disappear for an hour or so on a brisk walk, sometimes without breakfast, but always with a snack in my pocket in case of emergency. Three or four miles later I would return ready and able to eat a hearty protein filled lunch with my internal balance restored.

This became the established pattern for Christmas for the next fifty odd years. Now, at this present day, due to circulatory and heart conditions arising from living with diabetes for sixty years, I have to observe strict restrictions on my carbohydrate intake and the resultant insulin adjustment that takes precedence. However by being sensible and careful, the various treats of the Christmas season can still be enjoyed. Having said this I would like to see again a bar of the diabetic chocolate made with the formula used back in 1951.

Once again I would emphasise that people like myself with this condition should use common sense in the restriction of their carbohydrate intake, adjustment of insulin and exercise. Like myself you all have the ability to master this condition and gain knowledge from your own experiences. Never shirk from the challenges you will face and do not use diabetes as an excuse for not experiencing or enjoying the things that others take for granted. I would say "go for it"; I did and I have had a great life.

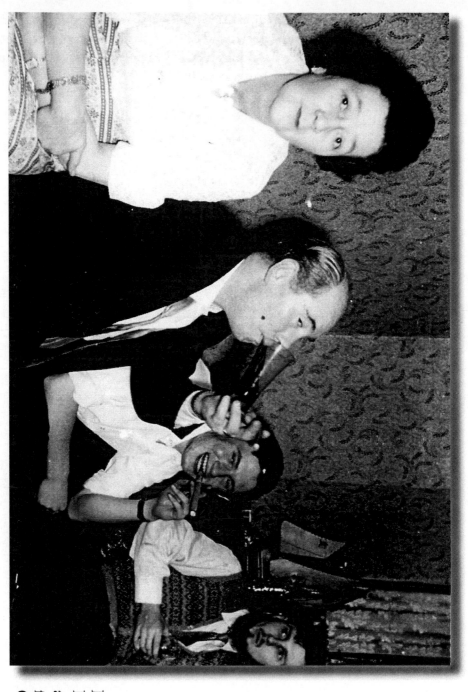

Mum and
Dad, John
and Alan in
front room
Cator Street

Adolescent Years

The time had finally arrived for me to return to school. The teachers had very little, if any, knowledge about my medical condition or its possible ramifications so I had to take it upon myself to explain as much as I could, with the possible exception of the P.E. master. This development with myself caused them no problems and it did have one pronounced advantage for me. I was now far less frequently on the receiving end of the hurled blackboard duster. However I was way behind with my school work having missed the past nine weeks of school with the result that at the end of my first year at senior school I was downgraded to class 2B1.

Never a fan of team sports and with no great enthusiasm for gymnastics my one real interest in the physical activities available at school was swimming. It was this, with the added danger of exercise in water, that caused the P.E. master concern. His concern, however, was eventually overcome by a letter from my parents after my father, together with a group of his friends, had taken me for two hour swimming sessions on Sunday mornings in the local pool. After about four or five of these sessions I always appeared to be less tired than any of the adults who would, each in turn, habitually challenge me to race lengths of the pool. The P.E. master subsequently relaxed his objections to some degree.

With the team sports, either football or cricket which we occasionally played between classes at a local park, I would always insist on being placed in a position which would require the least running about, i.e. in goal or the outfield. This enabled me to frequently slope off to the edge of one of the two ponds in the park where I would watch the ducks and voles or check for frog, toad or newt spawn all of which could be found there in the spring.

Prior to September I had enjoyed playing cricket with two or three of my friends using the lamppost outside the house as a wicket. I enjoyed it even more when my father managed to acquire for me an old cricket bat and a proper cricket ball from one of his acquaintances. On numerous occasions, after one or other of us had hit the ball it had the unfortunate habit of making contact with a neighbour's window following which the perpetrator, not myself I might add, would invariably drop the bat indicating his innocence! Sadly, however, on one such occasion that person dropped the bat and in triumph took a celebratory swing round the cast iron lamppost, caught his heel on the kerb and smashed his face against the lamppost. My father instantly ordered a stop to our cricket games in that particular location but the alternative, i.e. the area of park on which our P.E. lessons took place, was far too large for my liking.

It was whilst playing one of these games on what had just a few minutes before been a beautiful bright and sunny day that I witnessed one of the most incredible sights I have ever seen. The sky suddenly became very dark and there was a tremendous crash of thunder followed by very impressive sheets of lightening. We three pre-teen lads squeezed into the small porch that encased our front door and watched in incredulity as a line appeared in the middle of the street. On the opposite side from us the rain was bouncing about six inches off the pavement but on our side it was bone dry, a circumstance which persisted for some minutes. During my lifetime I have witnessed many different sights and aspects of the U.K. in its full and diverse range of weather conditions over all sorts of terrain from one side of the country to the other, with the exception of Ireland, but never have I ever seen anything to compare with the amazing spectacle of that day and in, of all places, South East London.

Perhaps because of my predilection for assuming the position of goal keeper in the game of football, one of my classmates, Peter Duen by name, would, on a number of occasions, initiate a brawl with me. He was shorter than myself but very fast and accurate with his punches, particularly aimed at the kidneys. With my reliance on insulin the last thing I could afford was sustained and concentrated energy output since if I fell down with a hypo I would be completely at his mercy. So, on the first two occasions he started a brawl with me I took a real hammering. On the third such occasion, however, by pure mischance, with the others as usual yelling "fight" and crowding round, he came fast at me but came into full contact with my head as I was ducking down and backing away. As a consequence Pete ended up in a heap on the floor with blood streaming from his nose, having been an unintentional victim of what I was later to learn was known as the "Glasgow kiss". Other than that one individual my relationship with my other classmates and teachers was quite cordial and my diabetes caused me few problems.

There was one incident, however, that indirectly caused myself and Alan great amusement. Whilst walking back to school after lunch one afternoon we stopped and went into the B.H.S. store in Rye Lane. Alan wanted to buy what he always referred to as "nutty", having picked up a lot of his elder brother's naval slang, which, translated, meant "sweets". Obviously because of my diabetes I was not allowed to have anything like that so I decided to buy half a pound of carrots.

Having paid for our purchases at the counter where the items were displayed, as in those days was the practise, we mooched around the store for a few more minutes before resuming our journey back to school. As we were leaving, myself with the carrots I had bought making a distinct bulge in my pockets, I was suddenly brought to an abrupt halt by a firm hand on my shoulder. On turning round I was confronted by a thick set man some eight inches taller than myself who demanded to know what was in my pockets. When I told him he clearly did not believe me and I was brusquely told to empty my pockets and place the contents onto the pavement at his feet. The thought immediately crossed my mind that when supplied with the evidence that I was indeed telling the truth it was conceivable that the man, as his manner suggested to me, would spitefully trample the carrots underfoot. I therefore declined his instruction and asked him by what right he thought he could make such a demand.

He adopted an even more menacing attitude and said he was the store detective and it was his belief that I had been shoplifting inside the store and unless I obeyed him I would find myself in very deep trouble. His demeanour made me think that perhaps I should do as he demanded so I reluctantly reached into my trouser pockets and produced a handkerchief, a couple of pence in change, two barley sugars and a rabbit's foot which I placed on the floor as instructed, then innocently looked up at the man towering over me. His immediate response was to accuse me of being a comedian and barked at me to also empty my blazer pockets. This I duly did laying at his feet a pencil, rubber, six inch ruler and a tattered notebook from an inside pocket. This produced an indignant scowl and he again seized my shoulder with one hand whilst thrusting his other hand into my outside blazer pocket. Upon withdrawing a handful of small carrots from this and also the remaining pocket a look of intense rage crossed his face. In a somewhat more subdued manner he told me to stay where I was while he checked that the carrots had been paid for. When he returned he told me that the assistant had confirmed the purchase because she particularly remembered me asking her not to put the carrots into a paper bag. They were both intrigued to know why I had requested this and I explained that if I returned to class with a paper bag it would have been confiscated and as I could not eat sweets due to my condition I would munch the occasional raw carrot. The barley sugars were, in essence, emergency medication.

Having listened to my explanation the store detective apologised to me with a mortified expression on his face for the way he had treated me. However he advised that in future it would be better if I agreed to my purchases being put into a paper bag which I could throw away moving the contents to my pockets once I had left the store. That way I would not arouse anyone's suspicions. Furthermore if I arrived back at school late then I was to ask my teacher to contact the store and they would explain what had happened. In the event this was not necessary as Alan and I, endeavouring to control our laughter, rushed back to school and managed to get there just as the last of our colleagues were entering the building.

Once again I had challenged what I had considered to be an unjustified and heavy-handed attempt to exercise power and authority over me. In the eyes of many adults I was a bumptious, over confident and cocky child without any perception of positions of power. However unless that power was used with fairness, logic and common sense the absence of one or all of these qualities would promote in me a sense of challenge which I would invariably accept and rise to meet.

On completion of the second year at the Adey's Road section of the school we all assembled, following the summer holiday break, at the Chourmert Road site. During that holiday Alan and I had hatched a plan between us to walk down to the Wye Valley if I could persuade my parents to allow me to take a holiday on my own rather than accompany them for the usual family fortnight at Ramsgate. Now at the age of fourteen and having to some degree reassured my mother, who would always ask me for guidance on how much of the various foods I could eat, that I was capable of looking after myself in that respect, she reluctantly agreed.

However there was still the hurdle of persuading my father to agree to my request. With his lorry driver's experience I was anticipating his objections to his son hitchhiking and youth hostelling. To my surprise and delight he also reluctantly agreed. He was aware that like himself at around the same age, his eldest son was beginning to feel the urge to find his own feet in the world and venture away from the security of the family environment. He was a little disappointed that in my case this urge had occurred at the tender age of fourteen but he offered me sound tactical and safety advice on the do's and don't of securing lifts and even arranged for one of his colleagues to convey Alan and myself to Gloucester on the first stage of our journey.

When we had seen and examined the cathedral at Gloucester and the remains of Tintern Abbey, enthused by them we amended our plans and decided to add the cathedrals of Bristol, Wells, Salisbury and, if possible, Bath to our itinerary. All these visits were accomplished with no significant problems on the diabetic front aside from the occasional need for barley sugars.

The cathedrals were a joy for us and Alan had sensibly managed to borrow a pair of binoculars from one of his brothers. These enabled us to gaze in wonder at the medieval skill and craftsmanship and the artistry of the beautiful stained glass windows, particularly those on the west front of Wells cathedral, which impressed us tremendously.

Confronted with this man-made beauty and the glory of the countryside between each location both myself and Alan were dumbfounded at the sheer stupidity of mankind who, over the past fifty years, had been doing its utmost to destroy this heritage through two world wars, that our forefathers had left us hundreds of years previously.

This feeling was further advanced and confirmed when, on hitching between Bath and Salisbury, we were picked up by what I initially thought was a sports car but when the driver got out and beckoned us over, swung his driver seat forward and directed us to a rear bench seat. The back packs we carried were only lightweight, ex forces issue, that had been purchased in surplus stores which, in the early 1950s, were plentiful, particularly the store in Deptford High Street where I later purchased my first pair of denim jeans, a style I now favour even though I am now in my seventies.

Our back packs contained a light cotton envelope that was long enough to accommodate our bodies with a pocket at the top for a pillow. These were a YHA requirement that enables your body to be kept separate from the bed linen and blankets supplied for use on the bunks in the hostel. Our packs also contained a towel, change of shirt and underclothes, socks, a light weight sweater and trousers in case it turned cold, a one pint ex-service water bottle and food for lunch and would fit comfortably on our laps. Seeing that we only carried such small packs the driver had decided he could accommodate us in his car so had therefore stopped to offer us a lift. He asked us where we were heading and offered to take us as far as Amesbury. The driver and his companion, who was slighter in stature, the driver being thick set and heavy in build with a quite menacing look, were both dressed in loud check suites and were bound for Newbury races. If they were to make it in time they could only take us as far as Amesbury.

We were motioned to get into the car which was a Citroen DS19, newly introduced and purchased in France. However as we climbed in we were both disconcerted to see, lying on the rear parcel shelf, a long double barrelled shotgun. As we drove I noticed that the driver continually flexed his shoulders up, down, backwards and forwards in a seemingly nervous habit. I must admit that I did find this somewhat unnerving being used as I was to seeing my father handle a large eight wheel lorry, frequently hauling a trailer behind, with no unnecessary body movements apart from hand signals or when changing gear. The driver seemed to be not only unsettled but he drove extremely fast. Suddenly, to my utter amazement, his left shoulder dipped in a flexing motion and I caught a glimpse of the speedometer which clearly indicated we were speeding across Salisbury Plain at 100 mph! When, by way of a question, I pointed this out to him he asked me what age I was. Upon my response he said "that will give you something to boast to your mates about that at fourteen you have done a ton"!

Not long after this, upon seeing some mud on the road ahead, the driver turned to his companion and muttered "bloody Kate's been playing with their tanks again; too much of this and we're going to be late", and Alan and I looked in horror at the state of the heath on either side of the road. We were dropped off just outside Amesbury and with our thanks and their best wishes the car's occupants drove off. Alan and I spent some time speculating whether they were Bookmakers or, in view of the gun in the back of their fast car, possibly crooks, although they had been perfectly amiable towards us even though they both had a menacing demeanour.

Shortly afterwards, during our second lift of the day, we were given a lift into Salisbury in, of all things, a Rolls Royce limousine that was driven by an elderly man whom, his wife informed us, was a former general.

Having explored the sites of Salisbury – Old Sarum and Stonehenge, we headed back home footsore but well content. I had also managed, without mishap, with no scales and reasonable urine sugar tests to avoid any problems and reassure everyone that I could cope with the diabetes and get on with leading as normal a life as possible.

At the end of the summer break we returned to school at the start of our final year. It was 1952 and although rationing had not yet been lifted it was starting to be relaxed which meant that buying food and clothing was becoming easier. My school blazer was by now far too short for me and the elbows had been patched with rexine that many times that the material was now very thin so my mother had to consider the cost of replacing it. I suggested that she might like to consider getting a former RAF battledress jacket which could be suitably adjusted to the right size and onto which she could sew the school badge from my outgrown blazer. This would not only be more durable but would be far more comfortable for me and be a much better, longer lasting purchase. She, rather sceptically, agreed.

On our first day back after the holidays we all gathered on the tarmac area around the school where, looking south east, we could see a large area of smoke that was beginning to darken the sky. For probably the first and only time in our school career many of us willingly rushed inside where we climbed the narrow stone staircase leading to the third floor, pouring into whatever open rooms we could find. Once inside we all peered out at this anomaly and to the amazement and amusement of some of the watching throng discovered that the roof of the school building we had only recently vacated was ablaze from end to end. It fortunately transpired that nobody had been injured but the extensive fire and water damage had rendered the upper floor unusable.

This would have the result of a considerable increase in class size, together with other suitable adjustments, to ensure that the boys due to be admitted for their first term at senior school could be accommodated. These factors, taken together with the end of term examination results, meant that I started my final year as a member of form 3C1 and acquired three new friends with whom, over the course of the next thirty years, I was to share many memorable experiences.

It was during that first week of my final year that my next brush with authority occurred. One morning during assembly, as was my usual practice when the Lords Prayer was being said and the hands of all my colleagues were firmly clamped together, their eyes closed in prayer, my hands would either be hanging by my sides or held behind my back. The Master taking the service that morning drew this to the Head's attention as his previous attempts to reprimand me for this practise had all been unsuccessful. The Head Master summoned me to the stage in front of the assembled school where he proceeded to use me as an example of bad appearance which was not acceptable at his school. Starting at the top of my head he drew attention to my long wavy hair which, in later years, the females of my acquaintance confirmed was my most attractive feature, pointing out that it needed cutting. Additionally my tie was worn at "half mast", my jacket was not suitable as school uniform despite the school badge and my shoes were badly in need of polish.   Finally, in an undertone, he told me to present myself in his office after assembly and dismissed me from the stage re-emphasising his previous remarks. He then proceeded to close the morning's assembly.

The boys broke ranks and wandered off in the direction of their respective classes and being one of the few remaining in the hall I started to follow my class mates. The Head Master caught my eye and waving his hand to the rear beckoned for me to follow him. He had a final word with the teacher who had brought me to his attention then left the hall. I followed him into his office where he indicated that I should take a seat on a chair that was placed at the front of his desk. As I pulled the chair further back to allow myself enough room to sit comfortably I noticed a framed photograph of a woman and two girls. From the clothing they were wearing I guessed that it had probably been taken in the early 1930s and estimated that the Head Master must be around fifty five years of age. As he sat down he told me he had been a Japanese prisoner of war following the fall of Singapore and asked me if I had any idea how such prisoners had been treated. I responded that I had read some accounts and overheard comments made by adults on the subject in the years since 1945. He said it was his firm belief that it had been his faith and belief in the Almighty that had brought him through that terrible experience and that, knowing what had happened in my life over the past two years, he was sure the Lord had intervened on my behalf and would like me to open up to that. He smiled at me and waved for me to leave the room but when I hesitated asked if there was something I wanted to say with an expression on his face which suggested that he clearly expected me to agree with him. In the event, however, he was due to be disappointed. I asked him if the photograph on his desk was of his wife and children to which he nodded that it was. I then asked him if it was not his love for them and his determination to see them again that had brought him through. In my own case it was the knowledge and dedication of a doctor, who himself had diabetes, that had saved me. It was now up to me to control my condition. He smiled and confirmed that all I had said had indeed been true but a little outside help now and then could prove useful. He then wished me a good final year in school and told me if I had any problems I was not to hesitate to contact him and it was now time for me to return to my class.

I can honestly say that I did knuckle down and try to reach a reasonable standard of achievement that year and the diabetes just became my normal way of life. By this time my mother had taken on an early morning cleaning job which meant she had to leave the house by about 7.45 a.m. My mother had purchased a small porridge cooker which was basically a container into which she put a mixture of oats and water which was then put inside another container of water with a lid over the two; this she would then put onto the stove and on her way out yell up the stairs for me to get up then leave for work. The porridge was then my responsibility.

After testing and injecting myself I would make a pot of tea, call my brother and sister to get up, make my sandwiches and oversee breakfast. I would divide the porridge up into three equal parts putting some salt into my share. After adding a dessertspoon of sugar I would then return the rest to the porridge container on the stove, i.e. Colleen's and Len's share, invariably having to call them again to get up. We all usually left the house together with Colleen accompanying her younger brother to his school then carrying on to her own. Out of the three of us I had the longest journey and would set off from the bottom of the street in the opposite direction.

I am frequently told nowadays by medics that given the duration of my diabetic condition I must have been blessed with good genes. However I must also have a few dodgy ones because I was constantly being told as a youngster to stand up straight and pull my shoulders back. Indeed at one stage when I was about nine years old consideration was given to fitting me with a back brace but due to a tendency to bronchitis, which I always contracted for a least a fortnight during the winter months until I moved out of London in 1961, this was felt not to be appropriate. As a result, at that time, I had to time to rely on physiotherapy and constant instruction from my parents and teachers, my father in particular, to correct my posture. My father was six feet tall, broad shouldered and ramrod straight but my maternal grandmother had a curvature of the spine which, in their later lives, was also inherited by her three children as it had in me. However my siblings and two out of every seven of those of my cousins whom I have seen over the last ten years or so appear to have escaped this genetic inheritance.

The other marked tendency I have is to wear down the outer edge of the heels of my shoes. This has been evident throughout my life as has a rolling gate when walking which enables me to be recognised from either a front or rear perspective long before people can see my face. I subsequently learned from an Orthopaedic Specialist that the angles to the assembly of the bones in my feet were outside the norm. Replacing the heels on my shoes was by far the best way to combat this problem. This diagnosis was given to me some time around the late 1980s when, following an operation on a carotid artery to clear cholesterol which may have been the cause of a stroke I had at the time, I had to have a number of MRI scans.

The one problem I had inherited from my father's side was sinusitis, possibly as a result of our so-called "retroussé" nose (i.e. upturned - generally small with a narrow bridge and turned up tip). In the 1950s, perhaps enhanced by the not infrequent London smogs, on many occasions I had to have my sinuses washed out. The method used was to sit me in a chair similar to the ones used by dentists and a hollow tube, approximately the diameter of a large biro, was introduced into one of my nostrils. Through this tube was inserted a solid rod with a point at one end and a hand grip at the other. The doctor would then place one hand at the top rear of my head which he would ease back against a headrest. With his other hand, using an occasional twisting motion, he would endeavour to force the rod up into the sinus cavity in the skull. During this procedure my hands would be firmly gripping the arms of the chair with my stomach muscles contracting even more firmly and I would desperately fight the urge to cry out in protest. After several minutes following this sustained pressure there would suddenly be a crack which would echo round my skull indicating that the rod had finally broken through into the sinus cavity. I would then be seized with a sudden fear that the force of the rod being thrust upwards like that would exit through the back of my head.

Having to sit through this on just one nostril was bad enough but there were a number of occasions on which the procedure had to be performed on both! Once breakthrough had been achieved a warm solution was then poured into the hollow tube to wash out the sinuses. This was by far the worst sensation I have ever experienced at the hands of a medical professional who was only trying to help me overcome any of the problems I had to endure. Mercifully, nowadays, I am told the technique has changed with either heat or power assisted tools having replaced the brute force used in those days. I sincerely hope this is true; not having needed such treatment for a long time now, I cannot verify this one way or the other.

Whilst on the subject of medical treatment, diabetics are often warned that open wounds will take longer to heal as a result of the elevated blood sugar levels in their system. This need not necessarily be the case. I have, myself, on a number of occasions sustained quite serious open wounds. The first of these was on my ankle at diagnosis which I have referred to previously. The second occasion occurred at school when I had opted at a handicraft lesson to make an aluminium fish slice for my mother (these implements were not available in the 1950s). As I was drilling holes into the metal the drill jammed causing the blade of the slice to spin round and catch me across the base of my left thumb folding back quite a large section of flesh. This wound was secured in place with a light bandage.

The third occasion was when my carotid artery was opened up from the top under my chin to the base of my neck and the final occasion occurred when I was standing on damp soil in the midst of a hypo and fell backwards through the rear wall of my greenhouse writhing about on the floor trying to take a box of glucose tablets out of my shirt pocket on broken glass. A surgeon had to remove a 30mm shard of broken glass from my left buttock. These last two instances required stitching and in the subsequent words of the medics "for an insulin dependant diabetic this has healed without any problem, far quicker than expected". This is what you too can achieve provided you follow a strict carbohydrate control, as I do.

Having now reached the age of fifteen and with the end of school approaching we were being advised that much would depend on our school testimonials which we would all receive at the end of term. These were currently in the course of preparation so we should all be on our very best behaviour during our last week as they could always be amended or even withheld if deemed necessary. So it was that on our final day we were first given the chance to say goodbye to our friends and also the teachers of the various subjects we had been taught and finally, before we departed, to collect our respective testimonials from the Head Master. When my turn came I entered Mr Wall's office and with a smile he handed me my certificate and said "I am sure you will do well in whatever you decide to do Tony but you will find it a lot easier if you become less inclined to challenge authority". He then shook my hand and offered belated apologies for having dressed me down in front of the assembled school two years earlier but with a final shot said "get your hair cut before you go for an interview". I decided that he was not such a bad guy after all. The testimonial, however, contained a slight barb in the tail as it read "A bright, willing, intelligent lad who works well when interested"!

A group of us made arrangements to return in the evening to take part in a table tennis competition and the school would remain open for that purpose with three tables, bats and balls being made available. So that night having initially walked home, done my injection and eaten my dinner I returned to school. At about 8.45 p.m. after playing a number of games and eventually being eliminated from the competition, I walked back home. My mother greeted me with "you timed that well, sit down and eat", with which she placed a plate of egg, bacon and a fried slice of bread in front of me. I just sat there looking at it and following constant urging from my father to eat he promptly picked me up off the stool and, with Colleen preceding him to open the kitchen and street doors, he carried me out to his truck. Once there he placed me between two rolls of tarpaulin on the truck's open back and drove me straight to the A&E department at Kings College Hospital. There I was swiftly given an injection of glucose and much to my father's relief soon recovered and was able to return home sitting by his side in the driver's cab of his truck.

This taught me another important lesson; sometimes, but not always, those nearest and dearest to you notice by various means that you are sinking into a hypo even though you may not be fully aware of this yourself. I would urge you to trust their judgement because they know you best. If it subsequently transpires they were mistaken you can always take exercise, reduce your next meal or adjust your insulin dose. However, as I have come to realise over long years of experience, it is usually the case that those closest to you who know you well are frequently correct in their judgement. Sometimes we who have this condition are so determined to master it that we either miss the signs altogether or ignore them.

When I was about ten or eleven years of age my father, who had been a shop steward, had been invited to attend a meeting of his fellow stewards in motor transport which was to be followed by a social evening for the families and he had taken my mother and us three children along. I had managed to surreptitiously slip into the room where the stewards were discussing the tactics they should adopt in order to pursue their objective of bringing about the nationalisation of the road transport industry. I was intrigued and fascinated to hear those men, my father prominent amongst them, analysing the potential advantages and disadvantages that success in this regard would bring not only to the drivers but also all others employed in that industry up and down the country.

At the end of the meeting, having reached a unanimous decision, they then proceeded to discuss the matter of nominating one of their number as a candidate for membership of the Executive Council of the Transport & General Workers Union (T.G.W.U.). I was absolutely delighted when my father was duly chosen to stand as representative for this position and let out a whoop of joy, and I guess triumph. With a huge grin the man in charge of the meeting said "well Len I hope the wife is as delighted as he is". This was a somewhat pertinent remark as my mother was not that pleased and I think this was the first time I had heard the term "black listed" used . My father was subsequently elected to the Executive Council of the T.G.W.U. and over the course of the next couple of years the road transport industry was nationalised with the eventual formation of the B.R.S. (British Road Services).

In the following years during the school holidays, half term breaks, etc., I would often accompany my father on his driving trips, becoming familiar with the glories of the British countryside and the seeming endless variety of different scenes it offered during all four seasons. During these trips I would often rest my head on a pillow placed on top of a folded blanket on the engine cover when I started to become a little drowsy where the steady throb of the diesel engine would lull me to sleep. When my father had had enough of sitting behind the enormous wheel of his truck we would occasionally spend the night at a house offering bed and breakfast accommodation to drivers. The various addresses of these houses would be exchanged between the drivers at transport cafes up and down the country where they would all inevitably stop for a break at some time or other in their driving schedules.

There was one thing about these B&Bs that really intrigued me; there would always be a large jug of water and a bowl placed on a small table near the bed. The first time I ever stayed in one of these houses it was with some surprise that I watched my father, when he got out of bed the next morning, pour some cold water into the bowl and from the small canvas sack he carried, take out a bar of soap, his shaving brush and razor and a small towel. Then, using only his huge hands, he would scoop up some water, thoroughly wet his face and torso, plunge his hands back into the water and work up a lather with the soap following which he would proceed to have a thorough wash, then take up his razor and shave. Having completed these administrations he would rinse off any soap suds remaining on his body and empty the water into the "jerry" under the bed. As he was drying himself off I would be instructed to clean my teeth then, with the remaining water, follow the same washing procedure, with the exception of course of shaving. Even in the height of summer, the water was never more than tepid and frequently, it seemed to me, ice cold.

Ablutions completed we would then go down to breakfast which usually consisted of a couple of kippers, a mug of tea and toast with either jam or marmalade. Following this my father would then roll himself a few cigarettes for the continuation of our journey, pay for the night's accommodation and meal and usually engage in a brief conversation with our hosts before resuming our journey. The various places we stayed at during these journeys always reminded me of the stagecoach depots that featured in the western films that were always being screened back then or their equivalent novels.

If my father ever under estimated the timing of these journeys it would usually be as a result of having to wait longer than anticipated for his truck to either be loaded or unloaded upon arrival at the designated destination. However, apart from the docks where there was strict demarcation of the dock workers, he would normally be actively involved in organising this himself. In the event he had no control of this then he would be driven to despair and despite everyone being members of the same trade union he was allowed to do no more than drive the unit to the designated points all of which were at different locations. All this mounted up to time delays when he was unable to perform his prime function which was to drive between points A and B. This sometimes caused him to lose his temper and spitting and cursing he would go in search of a foreman or shop steward best placed to overcome the hold up which would thereby enable him to get an infrequent opportunity to spend a night at home in his own bed. Looking back now, aside from the company I provided him with, which for my part I certainly enjoyed, I also wonder whether or not my occasional presence on these trips gave my father the opportunity of using me as a bargaining chip in getting himself moved up the queue whilst waiting for the dockers' attention.

Anyway, having again got underway, my father would, if he had no cigarettes already rolled up and the road ahead looked straight and clear, switch from heel to toe on the cab floor, clamp the steering wheel between his braced knees then, flexing his ankles rather than his wrists, proceed to roll himself a cigarette all the time holding the truck and trailer no more than six inches from the edge of the road. I would invariably be sitting on the left hand side of the cab with my head hanging out of the window on the few occasions I witnessed him doing this so I could clearly see the dexterity it took to hold such a large vehicle in this manner and I was incredulous at his driving skill.

In those days, of course, the volume of traffic on the roads was much lower than today and it a truck was approaching from the opposite direction it was not at all unusual for the drivers to recognise each other from either the livery on their trucks in the pre-BRS days, or from depot destination or number plate after the BRS had been established. Most of the drivers would drive resting their right arm on the open cab window, either out of habit or because the wind on their elbows kept them alert and the lower forearms of the heavy goods drivers were usually well tanned irrespective of the time of year. When passing another truck they would often yell in greeting to their counterpart by name, sometimes actually slapping hands as they passed as if they had known each other for a sufficient length of time to give them the confidence in each other's ability to carry out such a manoeuvre in complete safety.

These drivers also had a means of communicating with each other, day or night, by using hand signals or the lights on their trucks but rarely using their horns. In this way they could keep each other informed of may lay ahead of them on the road in front whether this was an accident, ice on the road, police diversion, etc., and each one had a separate signal code.

Unless we were likely to be home in time for dinner my father would usually pull his truck into a transport café where there would always be between twelve and twenty other drivers eating a hearty meal. A good half of these men would always greet my father by name and we would sit amongst them and enjoy a meal of eggs, bacon, sausage and a fried slice of bread. To the best of my recollection foods like chips, mushrooms or tomatoes, were not on offer in the late 1940s and probably due to the shortage of fats in those days, the fried bread was cooked using the melted fat from the bacon and sausages.

I can remember one particular day, when it was raining heavily and had been for some time, there were five of us sitting round the same table and in agreement with my father the other three declared that as the rain appeared to be countrywide there was no likelihood of them placing a racing bet that day. Like most of my father's close friends, they all liked to gamble. So the four of them each indicated and nominated a different raindrop on the rain streaked window and bet which one would reach the bottom of the window first. I just sat there open mouthed watching this spectacle, bemused at the strange ways of adults.

I think the thing that truly amazed me most was that no matter where we were as a family anywhere in the country, whether this was in Kent, Devon, or Essex, my father would frequently be greeted by, to me, complete strangers, and would engage in animated conversation for at least ten minutes. However, some twenty years later, this even happened to me when I believe I was in North Wales and had, for some reason, to give my name which was overheard by an elderly man. He caught my attention and asked me if I was related to Len Huzzey by any chance. Quite stupefied I replied that indeed I was, being his son. He then asked me to pass on his best wishes and assured me that my father was one of the best people he had ever met.

One day in 1951, when we were visiting the Festival of Britain site, and after my father had been stopped and greeted at least half a dozen times, I can remember my mother finally putting her foot down and saying "this is not fair on the children, there's a lot they want to see". Whether these frequent encounters were with other "knights of the road", as they were known then, or Trade Union buddies I do not know but one thing I know for sure is that my father made a lasting impression on an awful lot of people throughout his lifetime.

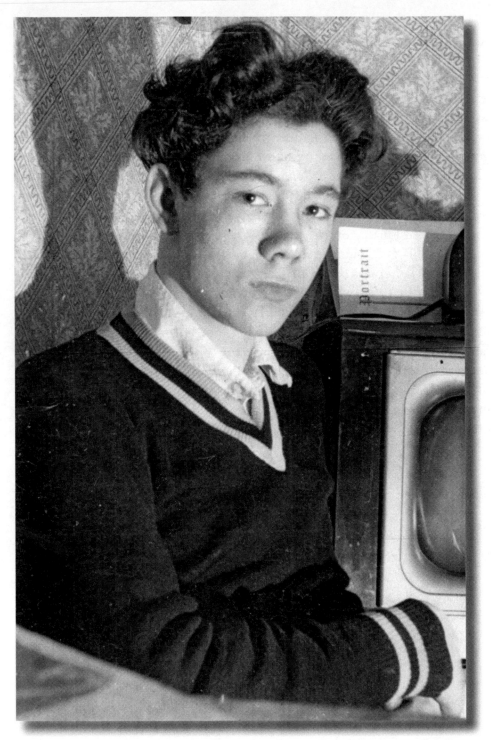

Aged 16 but still not following my Headmaster's instructions to get my hair cut

My Entry Into Working
Life & Trade Unionism

When we left school, Alan and myself had become increasingly concerned that there appeared to be no way that those of our generation could express our feelings with regard to world events, particularly since a Tory Government was again in office. This concern was prompted by events at that time such as the Yankse incident in China when the Chinese had opened fire on a British warship in the Yankse River, the issue of Indian independence, the ever increasing number of nuclear tests and the escalating conflict in Korea.

As a consequence we decided to make approaches to the local Labour Party to enquire if they had such a thing as a youth group. My father had been a member for quite a number of years and advised us that the Peckham branch was moribund and the local M.P., a woman named Freda Corbet, was reputed to have only ever asked one question in Parliament and that was just "can we please have a window opened because it is hot in here."! I am afraid that my father's cynicism was another trait of his that I inherited. He advised us that the East Dulwich branch would be a better option so, having established when and where they met, Alan and I went along one evening to one of their branch meetings. You can imagine the surprise that greeted two very young people that evening from the twenty or so silver haired people present who were only accustomed to meetings with people of their own generation.

As it turned out there was no youth group so we asked if we might be allowed to put forward a few of our ideas. This request was met with a great deal of scepticism but the Chair asked those present if they would be prepared to listen to these youngsters who had just appeared there that evening. Following some muted exchanges it was duly agreed that we be allowed ten minutes to introduce ourselves. We used this time to outline our concerns in relation to international and also domestic issues and requested assistance in the production of a leaflet we planned to distribute to our contemporaries in age. As expected, this gave rise to both observations of interest and also concern but the overriding consensus was that they had neither the time nor the resources to accede to such a request.

We left the meeting that evening obviously disappointed but not surprised at this reaction so we decided to do what we could ourselves. Alan was due to begin full time study so he would approach the Students Union at, I believe, the University College London, for assistance. I was also due to commence study at the Borough Polytechnic so decided to approach the Union. At that time, it was only us two among the five friends who had an abiding interest in politics. This was also, I suppose, my first attempt at becoming involved in organised and formalised politics which would later, as this account I hope will reveal, amount to something of use in the lives of my fellow citizens. This will be a decision I leave for yourselves to judge.

Over the course of its development mankind and evolution has developed many different modes and habits of living together but all ultimately have an inescapable link. Man is a social animal and ethnicity, nationality and religion are all concepts by which the animal has endeavoured to escape. The ultimate fact is, in common with all other forms of great ape, we are social beings who without that basic instinct would never have evolved to our current state. No one individual is more important than any other. The intellectual ability of each is basically potentially the same; it is circumstance which determines how that potential is either allowed or encouraged to develop. The current economic system which is predominately capitalism which at its core seeks to accumulate to the individual a greater share of resources than is available to another, has led to the degradation of the environment. The increasingly ominous likelihood of the potential destruction of the planet itself unless mankind rapidly wakes itself up and acknowledges the truth of John Ball's[1]

---

1   Little is known of Ball's early years. He lived in St Albans, Hertfordshire and subsequently at Colchester during the Black Death. He also lived in Kent at the time of 1381. What is recorded of his adult life comes from hostile sources liable to exaggerate his political and religious radicalism. He is said to have gained considerable fame as a roving preacher — a "hedge priest" without a parish or any cure linking him to the established order — by expounding the doctrines of John Wycliffe, and especially by his insistence on social equality. These utterances brought him into conflict with the Archbishop of Canterbury, and he was thrown in prison on three occasions. He also appears to have been excommunicated; owing to which, in 1366 it was forbidden to hear him preach.

These measures, however, did not moderate his opinions, nor diminish his popularity; his words had a considerable effect in fomenting a riot which broke out in June 1381. The chroniclers were convinced of widespread conspiracy implanted before the spontaneous uprising occurred, with the watchword "John the Miller grinds small, small, small" and the response "The King's son of heaven shall pay for all." Ball was in the archbishop's prison at Maidstone, Kent when the uprising began with protests in Dartford; he was quickly released by the Kentish rebels. He preached to them at Blackheath (the insurgents' gathering place near Greenwich) in an open-air sermon that included the following:

When Adam delved and Eve span, who was then the gentleman? From the beginning all men by nature were created alike, and our bondage or servitude came in by the unjust oppression of naughty men. For if God would have had any bondmen from the beginning, he would have appointed who should be bond, and who free. And therefore I exhort you to statement to the peasants' revolt in 1381:-

"Things will not be right until all is held in common".

As I am sitting here writing this account on the evening of 23rd October 2009, it has been announced that the economy is in its worst recession since 1955 and the announcer is querying why? To anyone with a grain of economic and political sense the reason is blatantly obvious. The so-called Labour Government some twenty years ago threw overboard the philosophy of its founding fathers and has now completely sold out to capitalism. When it was founded the aim of the Labour Party was to create a democratic socialist state. People like Kier Hardy, Ben Tillet and Annie Bessant must be turning in their graves. Fantastic levels of monetary resources have been poured into the support of an economic system which is corrupt to its core in both its policy and its operation!

Upon leaving school the immediate priority was to register with the Youth Employment Service and my initial contact with them was something of a disappointment. On announcing my intention of becoming an electrician it was suggested that my diabetes would hinder me in that ambition and I should be seeking something of a more sedentary nature. However if I was adamant then there was a post available with a radio connection, i.e. D.E.R.

In the early 1950s not many homes, other than the prefabs and newly erected blocks of flats that were being erected as the bomb sites were cleared, had electricity installed. The older housing stock that had survived the bombing or, like ours, had been patched up to make them habitable, relied on gas for lighting and cooking and coal for heating. The result of this was the infamous London "pea soup smogs". Therefore those houses without electric relied on an accumulator (wet cell batteries), a box of which could be used to switch between three or four channels, and a loudspeaker. The box, via an aerial, would receive a signal broadcast from a receiver in the area and when the signal became weak this was usually an indication that the accumulator needed recharging. There were a network of shops in most areas where people exchanged flat accumulators for charged ones.

---

consider that now the time is come, appointed to us by God, in which ye may (if ye will) cast off the yoke of bondage, and recover liberty.

Some sources, unsympathetic to Ball, assert that he urged his audience to kill the principal lords of the kingdom and the lawyers, and that he was afterwards among those who rushed into the Tower of London to seize Simon Sudbury, Archbishop of Canterbury. But Ball does not appear in most accounts after his speech at Blackheath. When the rebels had dispersed, Ball was taken prisoner at Coventry, given a trial in which, unlike most, he was permitted to speak, and hung, drawn and quartered in the presence of Richard II on July 15, 1381, his head subsequently stuck on a pike on London Bridge.

I was subsequently offered a job as an assistant at one of these receiver/transmitter depots in Peckham, about a one and a half mile walk from home. Here I found myself working in a dim and dingy basement without a breath of air alongside a man I would guess was around the same age as my grandfather. My job involved opening up the boxes, checking and cleaning the rotary switches for channel selection and checking and replacing any torn or split loudspeaker cloths. On very rare occasions I also soldered back broken connections. For this employment I was paid the princely sum of twenty two shillings per week (£1 and 10p in today's money).

I mastered all the above skills in my first week and my workmate, whom I discovered to be a pleasant, kindly old fellow, told me that I had mastered all this much quicker than any other youngster he had worked with before. He also said that there was no way I would be anything other than a wireman with that particular company and if I was indeed serious about being an electrician then I should look elsewhere. If I could walk there and back then I did not need to worry about the physical work and I was only a kid. He told me to find a job like this one when I had reached his age and was not capable of such physical exertion. With that sound advice I handed in my notice.

On my walks to and from work I had noticed a group of lads a little older than myself often gathered outside a small factory in a cul-de-sac known locally as the Melon Ground which was situated at the bottom of Rye Lane. Given that this location was very close to the end of the Surrey Union Canal it could possibly have, in the past, been the location of a dock receiving produce from the West Indies or Southern States of America. However that is pure speculation on my part for by the early 1950s, following the end of the war, the canal has passed out of use and is now a linear park.

Upon talking to this group of lads I discovered that the factory assembled and built fuse boards and switch gear and that it offered the opportunity to acquire some basic engineering skills. The starting wage was 40p a week more than I was receiving at D.E.R. and as it was closer to home and the employees there were mostly only a few years older than myself I sought and gained employment there. I was, however, disappointed to discover that this factory was a non-union workplace.

The small amount of money I earned at the job at the workshop, building switchgear, offered me the opportunity to purchase a new pushbike provided my father would agree to stand as guarantor for me to take out a hire purchase agreement. Following a lengthy lecture of the potential dangers to cyclists from motor traffic and the need to master manoeuvring the bike taking due account of traffic speed being far greater than mine, my father eventually agreed and I became the proud owner of a Raleigh Lenton sports cycle. Together with three of my friends, Ginge, John and Dave, we would often, in the evenings, cycle out to Richmond. I would have on me a pocket full of barley sugars, as cycling involves continuous and sustained exercise. On occasion, after I had taken the lead to set the pace, the other three soon became used to switching over positions whilst I fumbled with the paper encasing the sweet. I could usually succeed in popping it into my mouth as the third of my friends passed me, following which I would then resume my place at the front.

This became our established regime and, if we all felt up to it after reaching Richmond, we would, following a brief discussion, proceed to London Airport via Runneymead where we would spend twenty minutes watching the planes land and take off. One of our favourite aircrafts was the Lockhead Constellation, an aesthetically beautiful aircraft and the only passenger plane at that time to use tricycle undercarriage. In 1953 these arrivals and landings where from and to London Airport.

We would return home via a cycle path that ran parallel, but separate from, the road running alongside the Great West Road to Hammersmith. We would make our way through the traffic using side streets where possible to Camberwell Green. This was a twenty five mile journey and, excluding the twenty minutes spent at London Airport, would take us just over an hour. Over the following months we aimed to reduce this to under one hour and I am proud to say that after many attempts by honing our knowledge of various short cuts without reducing the twenty five miles measured by a mechanical counter mounted on the front wheel, our target was finally achieved.

Around this time I had struck up a friendly relationship with a chemist from whom I always got my supplies of needles and insulin and he drew my attention to two new products that had recently become available. The first of these was a Dextrose tablet about the diameter of a 2p coin and 7mm thick. These came in packs of ten and gave a more rapid release of glucose into the system than barley sugar.

The second product, and the first use of chemical technology in the treatment of diabetes that I can recall, was the Clinitest kit. This kit came in an oblong box that was split horizontally through the centre with the top half used as a container for the receipt of urine, the design of which I believe was appropriate for both sexes. The bottom half contained a small test tube, a rubber topped dropper and a bottle of tablets. The whole assembly was approximately 150 x 40mm.

The procedure for using this kit consisted of placing five drops of urine with ten of water together with one of the tablets into the test tube. Chemical reaction did the rest. To me, aside from the disposable syringe, this simple kit was by far the one and only advance, from the patient's point of view, that truly made life and living with the condition that much easier than had previously been the case.

By working the occasional Saturday morning I finally paid off the loan for the bike but, as I and my three friends soon realised our current bikes did not measure up to the designation of racing bikes. The main problem with mine was the three speed hub mounted Sturmey Archer gear. Given my height, by now over six feet, the handle bar post was too short so we now began to modify our respective "steeds". The first modification I attempted was to fit a four inch handlebar extension post thereby extending the handlebars over the centre of the front wheel. This allowed me to adopt a lower profile along the top of the bike.

The second modification I carried out followed as a consequence of an incident which still makes me wince at the memory. I had for some time been experiencing trouble with the S.A. gear which either kept slipping or locking. No amount of adjustment or lubrication would overcome this problem and one day when I put pressure on the right hand pedal as I reached the base of a humped back bridge over a canal to begin the climb, the gear slipped and I was thrown forward resulting in a very tender part of my anatomy coming into contact with the stem of the handlebar. This happened yet again as I reached the top of the bridge. Doubled up in pain, spitting and cursing I removed the back wheel and having jumped on it a few times to ease my aching groin I removed the tyre and inner tube, lifted the wheel above my head and, to the jeers and laughter of my friends, hurled it into the canal. For the second time in three years, this time with a bike across my shoulders, I made an uncomfortable journey from that bridge to my home albeit this time without the need to constantly stop, beg for cups of water or wetting myself.

At about the same time as this incident occurred I was sitting at home one night flipping through the jobs pages of my father's Evening Standard when my eye was caught by an advertisement for a trainee tea taster. Given that I did not smoke and, because of my diabetes, was precluded from eating sweet foots, I thought I might qualify so applied for my third job since leaving school. This resulted in me being taken on just before my sixteenth birthday by David Griegs, a grocery chain of mid market standing specialising in pork products and "up-market" teas.

My main task involved placing a small quantity of between twelve and thirty different types of tea into a small bowl, making an infusion of each in another then straining it off into a third bowl for the taster and blender to pass along in turn smelling, tasting and ejecting each one. With his deliberation complete he would make his choice of which varieties would be used to make up the different blends that the company sold. When this procedure had been completed, usually between 10.00 a.m. and 12.30 p.m., it was then my task to clear away, wash and dry the crockery prior to the whole process being repeated the following morning.

It always seemed to transpire that whilst I was up to my elbows in a large Belfast sink overflowing with suds and the jangle of crockery, the office door would open and one of the three post girls, who were frequent visitors, would enter. As a sixteen year old male I was not too disconcerted at this until one of the three, a tall brunette, Leanne by name, left me feeling acutely embarrassed and self aware. After about a month or so I had plucked up enough courage to ask her out for a date. We did indeed go out together a few times but sadly my first dating experience only lasted for about two or three weeks.

It had subsequently come to my attention that on the site of the shop and pork processing plant attached to it the resident maintenance electrician needed a mate. As I had never at any stage been asked to train in any of the steps the tea taster performed it was unlikely that I would make any progress in becoming a taster blender. With his reluctant agreement, therefore, I transferred to become the spark's mate in pursuance of my original ambition of becoming an electrician.

His role and responsibilities would often take us into the meat processing unit where I would watch in fascination as beef and pork carcases were brought in. The beef would be split into two halves lengthwise initially using a two-handed saw before being parted completely with a mighty blow with a razor sharp axe. A similar axe would be used to behead the pigs before they were cleaved end to end with the separated sections then proceeding on to the skilled butchers who would reduce the halves to joints and remove any offal etc. They would do this with the skilful use of knives, axes and cleavers of terrifying sharpness. On one of the few powered machines in the plant, the useful portions of offal would be used in the production of sausages and it was these machines which usually warranted our attention. There was obviously an overpowering smell of blood in this area but surprisingly very little sign of the liquid itself. It was the habit of the company to offer its employees a pound of meat of their choice from the offal or sausage range.

One Friday morning we found ourselves in the main shop of the company's premier outlet which was situated on the Waterloo Road adjacent to the Old Vic Theatre. The glass shades over the tubular pendant drops badly needed cleaning in order for the product lines, which were pitifully few in those days, to be seen clearly and to best advantage. These glass shades weighed in the order of two and a half kilos each and were secured by three small screws around the rim, suspended about ten feet (three metres) off the highly polished timber floor. By late afternoon, having successfully completed this task, alternating the cleaning and replacement of the shades between us using a three metre pair of wooden steps, we finally came to the last row of three fittings. Access to these had to be gained by positioning the steps between the sides and two ends of the meat counter. It being my turn to remove and replace the shades, I accomplished the operation on the first two, as I had successfully done throughout the day, but on reaching the last one as I tightened the third screw and released my supporting hand the shade crashed to the floor shattering into thousands of shards. In those days there were no refrigerated covered counters and the meat was on open display. The whole of the meat counter had to be cleared and scraped because of the possibility that bits of broken glass may have penetrated and contaminated the meat it contained. I was, as a consequence, not a popular lad since in the absence of refrigerated display cabinets in the mid 1950s, any unsold meat remaining at closing time would be shared amongst the staff.

As I said previously, our responsibility was purely electrical maintenance; any new installation work was carried out by a separate contractor. As it happened there was such an individual employed on the site who, after observing me working alongside the resident spark, offered me a job promising he would teach me the trade but with a higher wage than I was currently earning. Despite the spark's warning I was obviously tempted by the prospect of a higher wage and, what appeared to be, better training so I did indeed take him up on the job offer. However, on more than one occasion, this job involved me having to carry very heavy and awkward equipment on my bike. This was soon brought to the attention of my father by one of his colleagues who happened to catch site of me on an occasion when the sheer weight of carrying cable drums across the handlebars caused the bike's front wheel to get stuck between a tram line. All the time I was struggling to disengage the bike, which was well and truly stuck, from this unfortunate predicament there was traffic constantly passing on either side of me.

Not surprisingly, when he learned of this, my father was, to say the least, not very happy. He immediately stormed off to confront my erstwhile employer where he lived at the bottom end of Cator Street and proceeded to give him a real verbal tongue lashing for expecting me to undertake this kind of dangerous practice. Obviously quite intimidated by this confrontation, my employer handed over two week's wages on the understanding I would quit the job. In those days, both employers and employees in the building trade were only required to give or receive an hour's notice so the fact that I had actually received two weeks' wages led me to assume that my father must have scared the living daylights out of my employer.

When he arrived back home my father told me that the guy was no more than a "bucket shop operator" and if I really wanted to become an electrician then an apprenticeship was the only, and indeed the best, way of achieving this. He told me that one of his lunch time drinking friends, Albert, was a charge hand electrician and if I wanted him to he would ask him to enquire whether the firm he worked for would be prepared to take me on.

This subsequently led to an interview being arranged with the Managing Director of quite a large electrical contracting company at their offices in Vincent Square, SW1. My father accompanied me to this meeting where we ushered in to an imposing timber panelled office. Here we were met by a silver haired gentleman sitting behind a large heavy desk. He was about ten years older than my father and introduced himself as Mr V.S. Stock who was not only the Managing Director but also Chair of the N.F.E.A., the Employers' Federation. He patiently listened to an account of my employment history to date and went on to ask me some questions on my relative experience and my diabetes. He further questioned me on my ability to cope with the physical exertion that was part and parcel of a spark's working commitment and environment. I immediately recalled the response I had given to the Youth Employment Clerk some eighteen months previously when faced with a similar question and indignantly pointed out that I had cycled twenty miles at least two or three evenings every week. He asked me if, in that case, I would be willing to attend polytechnic college which may involve some evening classes. I replied that I would in the previous knowledge that I would be entitled to day release to attend college if I signed up.

On that basis Mr Stock proposed that I undertake an initial two month probationary period upon completion of which if I successfully met the company's expectations then I would be offered a four year indentured apprenticeship on my seventeenth birthday. He stressed to me that as the age for apprentices to sign indentures was normally fifteen and as I was already nearly seventeen then I would really need to knuckle down and prove my worth. As we left the building my father told me that he thought I had handled the whole interview quite well observing that the Managing Director had given me a very thorough grilling. He earnestly entreated me not to let either him or myself down.

On my very first day I was able to demonstrate there were very few items in the stores, including the most frequently used cable sizes, that I could not identify. I had also been able to further prove my knowledge retention when challenged to put a thread on the end of a piece of three quarter inch conduit I had been asked to cut and queried if that would be a normal thread or a runner, which was five times the length of a normal thread.

So, four weeks later, having successfully concluded my probationary period, I found myself, together with my father, again assembled in Mr Stock's office only this time with the inclusion of his secretary to witness our respective signatures. Mr Stock remarked his satisfaction that I had met the probationary requirements and arrangements had been made for me to attend the Borough Polytechnic. He told me that I now had the opportunity of acquiring both the practical and theoretical skills required of the job. This time as we left the building my father said to me "well done, now make sure that over the next four years you get your City and Guilds and become a first rate craftsman and teach that smug bastard a lesson".

That Friday afternoon, having signed my indentures, I was told to report the following Monday morning to the foreman at the firm's depot within Woolwich, Arsenal. After cycling down the hill in Woolwich, at the bottom of which stood the imposing arched gate to the Arsenal, and glancing to my right I could see the entrance to the Woolwich Barracks through which, in the late 1870s, my paternal grandfather had passed at the commencement of his military career. I was struck by the coincidence that both he and I, although separated by nearly eighty years, had started our respective careers in very close proximity to each other.

Upon arrival and after showing my letter of introduction to the guard on the gate, I made my way to the location he directed me to go. According to the distance counter attached to the front wheel of my bike, this was some third of a mile from the gate through which I had entered. My route took me past a number of large workshops from which emanated a variety of metallic scratching sounds. I had previously checked the distance counter on my bike after leaving home and it clearly indicated that my journey to work had covered a distance of six miles. The thought crossed my mind that when the weather turned rough it may not be as pleasant a ride as I had experienced that day.

However on proceeding through an ornate arched stone entrance to the depot's building with no visible notice to identify that I was in the correct location I was confronted by a large dim square area with the only light that was able to penetrate emanating through the archway. There being no-one in sight for me to ask for my bearings, I noticed an open staircase on the far wall which led to the floor above. On hearing muffled voices which I assumed were coming from this area I placed my bike against the wall inside the lower space and yelled "is this Berkeleys?" whereupon I received a response of "up here". I climbed the stairs and was confronted with a scene that was little different from that below except for the fact that this space contained a few extremely dirty rain streaked windows which at least let in a modicum of light.

At the end of the room stood a group of ten or twelve individuals listening to a fellow about the same height as myself but much stockier in build who looked to be in his late forties or early fifties. He beckoned for me to go forward and asked if I had a letter for him. I asked him in turn if he was the foreman of Berkeley Electrical Engineering and he nodded that he was. I then handed him my letter which he read and turning to the other lads said "OK, with the exception of you Paddy, the rest of you off to your jobs, this lad is our new apprentice and I will introduce you later". The foreman then turned back to me and asked me to further elaborate on the brief synopsis of my previous experience that had been outlined in the letter of introduction I had given to him which he had in turn passed to Paddy for his perusal.

After Paddy had read the letter the foreman said to him that it seemed I had already grasped and used the essential basics so he thought I should be given the chance to build on those by placing me with Eric and Ron on the crane gang where I would also gain some experience of Direct Current. He asked Paddy what he thought about that and Paddy agreed that it would certainly be a useful initial placement for me. The foreman turned to me and told me that Paddy was the shop steward and he would leave me with him for a while so that we could talk then after we had all had a cup of tea the foreman would take me down to the crane gang's depot where he would place me in Paddy's capable hands.

He asked me if I knew what the E.T.U. was and if I would consider joining. I responded that I had been trying to do so for the past two years but had been rejected initially due to the fact that the workplaces I had previously worked in were all unorganised. Although my last employer had claimed to be a member of the Peckham branch he had still refused my request for my name to be put forward for membership. At this I was asked for his name and my reply initiated a look of extreme annoyance on Paddy's face and he spat out "that bastard scab was expelled six months ago". Turning to me Paddy said "Tony, you will be welcomed with open arms into my branch, Central London No.2". So it was that a few days later I became a member of the Electrical Trades Union and a few weeks after that I became branch doorkeeper. It was quite often a source of amusement to those brothers present at future meetings that a mere seventeen year old would demand the production of membership cards to attendees I did not recognise in proof of their membership which would invariably be an adult far older and much heftier than myself.

It was perhaps this performance that influenced my persistent questioning of information and correspondence that came in from the Area or Head Office and my frequent participation in debates. Three months later, following the transfer of one of our branch members to another branch, I found myself elected onto the Branch Committee and, at my instigation, elected as delegate to the Southwark Trades Council and subsequently, eighteen months later, I was elected as Branch Chair. Central London No.2 was one of the most active branches in the London area; the area with the largest UK membership.

Some time after my election as Branch Chair I was appointed as a co-opted member of the 27 Area Committee in order to ensure the opportunity of a voice on behalf of apprentices when matters concerning them were on the Agenda. Although I had full rights to participate in discussions, as a co-opted member, I was not allowed to vote. However I was subsequently to use this opportunity to endeavour, successfully, to make sure that at the completion of their apprenticeships, every apprentice had achieved a good all round experience of the trade and were not treated as mere "tube hands" or "carcase kiddies".

It was whilst working on the crane gang that I encountered my first serious problem with diabetes. On a cold and frosty morning in mid February we were well into the refurbishment of a jib crane that was standing on the south bank of the Thames opposite the Ford plant at Dagenham. I had volunteered to go to the head of the jib to push a draw tape through the conduit we had previously replaced, into the cab where Eric would then attach it to the new cables ready for me to pull them to the top of the jib. So there I was, squatted at the end of the jib which was poised at a 45° angle some forty feet above the murky cold water of the Thames flowing beneath me and twenty five feet from the shore.

I had pulled the three cables about half way up when, with the effort involved in drawing them through, I began to feel tingling sensations in my hands. Despite the coldness of the steel girders on which I was sitting, I was beginning to sweat profusely and I knew only too well what these symptoms meant. This was not due to the effort involved in pulling up the cables but a sure sign I needed a barley sugar. Therefore I took off the gloves I was wearing and reached into my pocket to retrieve the sweet. However without the gloves I was struggling to remove the sweet paper wrapping with hands that were becoming colder and colder from the wind that was blowing up-stream from the estuary a few miles to the east.

Eric yelled up to me from the cab below to enquire if anything was wrong as I was no longer pulling up the cables. At this point Ron came out from the cab and looked up to my position where I had at last managed to unwrap the barley sugar and put it into my mouth. Realising things were not quite right he turned to Brian, the spark's mate, and told him that he had best go up to guide me down as I was obviously in trouble. If I missed my footing I would stand no chance of surviving such a fall. Brian immediately followed this instruction and helped me down and into the cab of the crane. Eric told us that was it for today and we should go back to the shack to warm up. He further went on to say that whilst I had told them what signs to look out for in relation to my condition they obviously needed further instruction so that would take care of the afternoon. The solidarity those lads displayed to me that morning instilled in me the importance of ensuring that my colleagues always knew how to deal with a diabetic reaction if I was unable to deal with it on my own.

However that was not to be the last of the day's incident. As I cycled the journey home at the end of the working day I was not relishing the climb up the hill on the route I had to take past the Arsenal gate so I decided to take an alternative, lower route, past Greenwich Naval College. Just outside the college was a row of bus stops and as I was cycling past, very close to the kerb, a bus began to overtake me. As it passed it clipped my right shoulder causing me to lean to my left. I then ricocheted from left to right down the length of all four buses parked there as I fought to stay upright. This was a very unpleasant experience.

The next morning I recounted this episode to my work colleagues and they suggested that as we all travelled from Peckham and there was a seat available in one of the two sidecars they used then it might be better if I used that method of transport instead of my bicycle, especially during the winter months. I consequently agreed to this sensible suggestion.

I spent the next six months working in a variety of locations in the Arsenal where I was continually fascinated by a wide range of heavy engineering practices and procedures. It seemed to me that much of this had changed very little since the dawn of the industrial revolution, except for the motive power supply. The most impressive was probably the site of a billet of red hot steel which would be slowly progressed through a direct current rather than water or steam powered hammer until it emerged as an octagonal four metre length of steel. When this cooled it was passed in turn to a huge lathe where a hole would be bored right through its full length. It would then proceed to a series of milling and slotting machines until it finally emerged fully formed as the barrel of a heavy gun. It would then be lifted clear of the machines, greased and placed on trestles to await its final destination mounted into either the turret of a tank or onto the carriage of a piece of field artillery.

Whilst I could not condone the thought of the death and destruction this implement would cause I was nevertheless full of admiration for the skill and expertise that had been used in its production by all those working class men who had converted a dining table sized lump of metal into the finished product. All this had been achieved working in conditions of very little light in either extreme heat or cold dependent upon the prevailing weather conditions at the time. The overall working environment could only be described as filthy and would, in my opinion, be exceedingly generous to describe them as primitive; appalling perhaps would be a more appropriate description.

It was now decided that in order to expand and enhance my position I should be transferred to a site on which I could remain from the setting of its foundations to it being handed over to the intended occupants. It subsequently transpired that this would be a school in Beckenham which was located a similar distance, now that I had resumed cycling to work, to my previous location. I certainly learned a great deal from this opportunity going right through the initial carcase, conduit installation then installation of the electrical wiring determining the circuitry to the final connecting up and commissioning.

Using the usual irreverent fashion of the nickname of sparks, and in recognition of how much I had learned and proved I was capable of, I was told to throw the main switch which would energise the whole installation. Looking at me the foreman said with a grin "OK Tony, let there be light" and in some trepidation I threw the main breaker and lo and behold there was indeed light. The school was now ready for the children to attend with no problems insofar as the electrical installation was concerned. The team of us who had all worked on the site duly departed in anticipation that perhaps some time in the future we may renew our acquaintance on another work location or it may be that we would never see each other again.

There was one other memorable event for me on this site. On arrival I discovered that although we were all "sparks", that is members of the E.T.U. (Electrical Trades Union), we were the only trade on the site without a steward. I therefore raised this with the lads with the suggestion that we hold a shop meeting to elect one of our number to that position. They were initially not keen on the idea since, at that time, particularly if there was either a personality clash with the foreman or any issue arising which could ultimately lead to industrial action, then any stewards would find themselves black listed with regard to further employment. However a meeting was duly held and somewhat to my surprise I found myself nominated for the position. I responded that if my colleagues were prepared to accept being represented by an eighteen year old apprentice then I would do it but I would need help and guidance since, although I had recently been elected as Branch Chair, there was a world of difference between the two posts.

The Scottish spark I was working with pointed out to those present that although he thought me an able and intelligent lad it would not be fair to put me in that position before I had completed my apprenticeship. Therefore it was up to one of them to volunteer since I was absolutely right in that they should have steward representation. One from our number was duly elected and to my surprise and delight would frequently engage me in quite lengthy discussions before raising any observations on working conditions or grievances with the site management. He would actively seek my ideas or suggestions on the appropriate action in raising or pursuing matters. This was a pattern that would re-occur throughout my working, and subsequent political, life.

Around this time I also attended a political education course at the E.T.U. college in Esher, Surrey. This establishment was located in a large pre-Victorian mansion which the union had acquired some years previously specifically for the purpose of educating its membership in the necessary skills to adequately train them for the role of representing their fellow workers and acquire an understanding into the interpretation of the economic and political implications of government or employer initiatives that may or could have on their working conditions or future prospects. Here we were trained in all the techniques required to defend and enhance the position of working people.

I eagerly participated in discussions which sometimes went on well after the afternoon lecture had finished ranging from 8.00 p.m. to well into the early hours of the following morning. The three lectures I attended covered the whole spectrum of left politics, right wing Labour to the Trotsky left.

I shared a room with another lad the same age as myself who, at the end of the course, suggested that if I wanted to enhance my political awareness then I might find it interesting to join a group that met in West Norwood who were led by a man named Gerry Healey. At the first meeting I attended I purchased a number of political tracts of Marx, Engels and Lenin. Some few weeks prior to this I had switched from buying my normal News Chronicle newspaper or

The Times which was then only published on Saturdays, to a daily publication – The Daily Worker.

Following further detailed discussions with both Alan and my father and my subsequent absorption and interpretation of Lenin's "Left Wing Communism, an Infantile Disorder", I made the decision to quit attending the West Norwood group which were to became the fledgling Socialist Labour League. Later, as is the habit of Trotskyite groups, they became The Workers' Revolutionary Party. Having looked into both militant and various other groups I decided I needed to join the organisation which seemed to me to be the most closely aligned with my own opinions and therefore became a member of the Young Communist League.

In the time that had elapsed since the problem I experienced with my diabetes on the crane incident at Woolwich Arsenal, nothing other than the occasional reaction I was able to overcome myself occurred. However it did cross my mind that I needed to lay down some ground rules to protect the safety of both myself and others around me as there would obviously be more occasions in the future when I would require the assistance of other people when I was subject to similar incidents. This decision was brought about because it was sometimes the case that during such incidents I would lose control of my limbs which would involuntarily lash out in all directions. It was also invariably the case that once sugar was placed into my mouth my subconscious reaction would be to spit it out in all directions. I therefore gave my friends and colleagues the following instructions should they be present when I was subject to these incidents. Firstly they needed to approach me with great care then after dissolving some sugar in water they should pinch my nostrils together and as my mouth dropped open to breathe slowly pour in this sweet liquid. They should then release my nostrils and placing a hand under my chin push upwards. This would subdue any subconscious attempt on my part to reject the sugar solution I needed. My subconscious automatically reacted in this way because under normal circumstances ingesting such a sweet solution would potentially result in me experiencing much more severe problems. I discovered that this simple strategy proved very useful in future years when, on a number of occasions, I was informed that during such episodes it had taken at least four or five people to hold me down and keep me still enough for one of them to administer the necessary sugar my body needed at that time to correct the problem.

With the relaxation of sweet rationing my favoured method of overcoming these reactions myself if I was able to was to make the experience an occasion to enjoy either a small bar of fruit and nut chocolate or, if available, a Pontefract cake or coconut cheesecake, all rare but very welcome treats.

One Saturday during this period of my life my friend Dave and I had decided to cycle all the way to Brighton which was about forty miles away, our other friends, Ginge and John, being otherwise engaged. Having dispensed with the gears on my bike I would make the trip riding with a fixed wheel which was great when riding on the flat or uphill but proved to be a bit of a problem when riding downhill. I either had to extract my feet from the toe clips and move my legs clear of the fast rotating pedals in order to protect my shins and calves from being struck, or keep my feet in the toe clips which meant pedalling furiously as the bike gathered speed in its descent. In the event I had no option but keep my feet in the toe clips and allow my legs to continue the very fast pedalling motion. As a consequence of such vigorous exercise and by the time we finally reached our destination, I had completely exhausted my supply of barley sugars and glucose tablets. This meant that I would need to inject prior to our return journey.

Having eaten and subsequently injected my usual dose of insulin and being unable to find anywhere from which I could buy more glucose tablets, I was not confident that the sweets I had bought would be sufficient to get me home, bearing in mind the experience of the outward journey. I decided it would be prudent to call into the A&E department at Brighton hospital and request a glass of glucose as insurance. With three years' experience my initiative told me this would be a wise move. Initially the medical staff at the hospital were sceptical of my request and reluctant to comply. However at the mention of the fact that I was being trained and advised by Dr Lawrence their attitude changed completely. So after swallowing a small glass of glucose Dave and I shaved ten minutes off the time of our outward journey and arrived home well satisfied with ourselves and without experiencing any untoward problems.

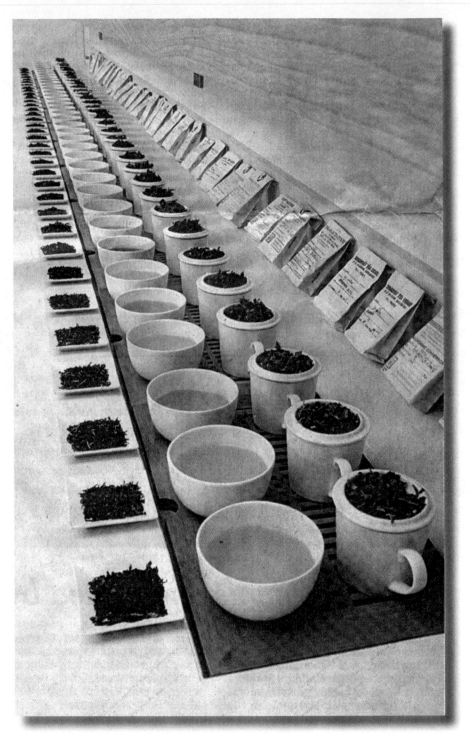

Typical layout prior to Tea Taster determining blends, these are the items I was washing up

Trades Union cards 1955 and 1959 from the start of my apprenticeship to its completion

Social Life and Completing Apprenticeship

Our eighteenth birthdays were now approaching and none of us lads had ever been particularly fashion conscious having no interest in the Teddy boy culture or the advent of rock and roll. Alan was now well into full time study and went on to achieve degrees in biology and education. Ginge, John and myself became avid trad jazz fans and Dave, the more conventional of the five, drifted off in pursuit of other interests. When each of us in turn was summoned to register for National Service, John was detailed to the R.A.F. and Ginge to the Royal Fusiliers where he saw active service in Aden. Alan was exempted pending completion of his degree and Dave was also exempted until he had completed his apprenticeship. With regard to myself, once I had proven my medical condition I was issued with a letter that I was required to produce if challenged. This letter stated that in the current circumstances, I was not required for service in H.M. forces. It occurred to me then, and even more so now, under what circumstances in a battle situation would a diabetic be able to inject and then, of necessity, eat?

As Ginge and John were soon to disappear off the scene at weekends, I began to develop the habit of meeting up on a Saturday night with two or three of my friends from the Borough Polytechnic, and go to the dance halls at either the Lyceum in the Strand or the Tottenham Royale. The lads with whom I had teamed up became regular readers of one or other of two journals I had been handing out to fellow students, initially prior to my leaving their group which were the Trotskyite "Keep Left" and subsequently the Y.C.L. youth magazine "Challenge". I was to discover later that this drew me to the attention of MI5. I had also become a regular reader of "Labour Monthly", a magazine of in-depth analysis of current, national, international, political and economic affairs. The editor, Rarji Palme Dutte, had a considerable international reputation as a left wing intellectual.

One Saturday night in September 1957, in view of the fact that two or three of us who frequented the dance halls and lived south of the Thames and the third in West Ham, we decided to add the Streatham Locarno to our list of venues. The reason for this was that the Royale was difficult for all of us to get to unless the lad from West Ham was able to borrow his elder brother's car. Additionally, until a recent hitch hiking holiday around Scotland with

Alan, I had also been seeing a girl at the Lyceum who lived in Wembley and although our relationship had been quite affable we had both subsequently agreed that as we lived so far apart we should both seek a friend closer to our respective locations.

On our first night out of London Alan and I, in quite appalling weather, had been dropped off in the middle of Sheffield with no hope of finding a youth hostel. We eventually sought the assistance of a policeman and suggested to him that perhaps we could spend a night in the cells. He laughingly rejected this suggestion and directed us to a nearby Salvation Army hostel with a few cautionary words of advice regarding our possessions. We reluctantly took his advice but were surprised to discover this was by no means as bad an experience as we had anticipated. However we resolved it was certainly not an experience we would wish to repeat.

Around five days and a host of varied lifts later, the most recent being on top of a sheeted trailer being towed by a farm tractor, we found ourselves at the top of a pass looking down into Glencoe. We had reached this point after walking about a mile from the point at which the farmer had dropped us off. With tears streaming down my cheeks I opened my mouth in awe at the shear beauty of the panorama spread out before us. To the left we could see water cascading down the steep sides of the Three Sisters, whilst to the right could be seen the even steeper slopes of the Chancellor Mountain and the breathtaking beauty of the Aonach Eagach, more commonly known as The Devil's Staircase. We watched in silence as the sun rose up the valley, bouncing off the gleaming surface of the waters of Loch Leven far below us.

The road we were on was enclosed by rough stone walls on either side to prevent traffic from straying off its twisted course and plunging deep into the valley below. Many years later I was to find myself the cause of concern to a coach party of Dutch tourists who were travelling along this same road and witnessed my endeavours to fit an air bag jack onto the exhaust of the car I was driving whilst trying to lift the caravan we were towing in order to change a wheel. Despite the contrast in scenery with that of Holland, for some reason they found my attempts with the air jack more interesting than the panorama stretching before them. This took place some thirty seven years after that first, never to be forgotten, sight of the majesty of Glencoe.

Having descended to the village, over the course of the following four days of incessant sunshine, Alan and I walked around Loch Leven and then half the length of Loch Ness. There was a youth hostel situated in the region of Urquhart Castle into which, on the evening of that fourth day, we eagerly booked accommodation. Being very hot and sticky I was desperate to go for a swim and not having seen any signs of the alleged monster of Loch Ness immediately discarded my haversack on the upper steel framed bunk of our pair, swiftly changed into my swimming trunks and without waiting for Alan dashed outside and along a short jetty from which I made a shallow dive into the cold water the shock of which hit with immediate effect onto my hot body. For the previous three days I had been continually sweating with the heat and exercise of walking and having swam about twenty metres under water rapidly returned to the jetty and hauled myself out. I stood there in the sun shivering violently having not given a moment's thought to the temperature of the water before I plunged in. Alan joined me grinning from ear to ear and told me that the lake was seven hundred feet deep so of course it was obviously going to be very cold. Very crestfallen I responded that I was now very well aware of that!

However that was to prove the least of my problems as I was soon to discover after returning to the hostel to get my towel. When I had thrown my haversack onto the bunk bed I had forgotten that I had wrapped my syringe and two vials of insulin inside my towel. This I discovered at my cost when I took it out from the bottom of my haversack and found to my horror on unrolling it, that all were now no more than broken shards of glass which had embedded themselves into an insulin dampened face flannel. This presented me with a severe problem and my first thought was to establish where the nearest G.P. was to be found so I contacted the warden of the hostel to make the relevant enquiries. Realising my predicament he eventually located and telephoned a G.P. whose practice was located some ten miles distant.

Three girls had also booked themselves into the hostel earlier in the day, one of whom happened to be a trainee nurse. At that time only youth hostels in Scotland accepted hostellers who used motor transport and fortunately for me she had a Morris Minor car parked outside. When the girls returned from their day's outing the warden approached the owner of the car and after explaining my predicament asked if she would kindly be able to drive me to the G.P.s' home.

On arrival the G.P. informed me that one of his patients was also a Type One diabetic whom he treated with bovine insulin[2]. He suggested that in

---

2   In the mid 1980s I believe the medical profession was induced by the pharmaceutical companies to throw overboard the regime of strict carbohydrate control that was initially taught to myself and others. The motivation for the drug companies to do this followed the discovery that by the manipulation of yeast and certain microorganisms they could produce, what they labelled "human insulin", at a far lower unit production cost than the purification process of producing insulin from either pigs or cattle. The philosophy behind this, in simple

terms, became "let them eat what they like and inject accordingly".

This led to three immediate consequences:-

1. lack of exercise;

2. industrial quantities of insulin being prescribed and injected as medics desperately tried to bring blood sugar levels under control, and multiple daily injections with the switch from urine to blood sugar testing. This obviously gave the drug companies an opportunity to generate even greater profits;

3. increased hospital admissions to A&E, including the time spent as admissions by individuals.

There are a multiplicity of blood testing machines now available, all requiring different lancets and test strips. None of them offer any perceptible advantage over the other and what difference does it make what colour meter you have or whether it gives a result in ten or four seconds? At the end of the day all this choice is only for the benefit of the drug companies to increase their profit margins.

In 1984 I proved the validity of the above assertions when, after failing to receive a response from the Department of Health (this prior to the Freedom of Information Act), I spent an hour with Robin Cook MP, the then Shadow Minister for Health, discussing with him the problem many of us were experiencing in using the so-called human insulin. As a result of his intervention the D.o.H. finally responded to my request for information. Their response bore out my suspicions that since its introduction the cost of filling insulin prescriptions had dramatically increased, as had both admissions to A&E and the number of nights spent in hospital as a result of diabetes.

In the early 1990s Tony Blair (who is not a politician I have much time for being myself a lifelong socialist) made an outrageous statement in Parliament that thousands of people in the UK owe their lives to the advent of human insulin. He either did not know or chose to ignore the fact (for reasons best known to himself) that since its discovery in Canada in 1922 animal insulins, taken in conjunction with a regime of strict carbohydrate control, had been in wide use throughout the developed world and had enabled many thousands of people to lead a useful and fulfilled life. What is more, following ten years of campaigning by a relatively small dedicated body of people, animal insulin is still available despite the fact that all the major drug companies have withdrawn it from their product lists.

During the course of the sixty years I have lived with this condition I for one am tired of hearing that things have improved. It is not true! Technology, together with specialist medical staff have been introduced and targets set for patients to achieve. However, insofar as the medical profession are concerned, I believe that paternalism reigns; the patient must be told what to do and must adhere to those instructions. Whilst this may be well meaning, I believe it is wrong. As Dr Lawrence told me sixty years ago, having to live in my body twenty four hours a day, I would become the expert. It was he who made it possible for myself and my contemporaries to receive an education in our condition and to manage and control it. He taught us to be independent and confident in our ability to do so, never allowing the condition to prevent us from doing all the physical things we wanted to do. We just needed to be self aware and to ensure we always have two barley sugars in our pockets.

The NHS now spends ten percent of its budget on diabetes. This, I believe, is out of all proportion. Of all chronic conditions diabetes is probably the easiest to live with. What needs to be done is to make sure that those newly diagnosed, particularly the young, are given comparable training to what I received in 1950 and encouraged, as I was then, to become order to overcome my immediate need I should go to the farm on which this female patient lived and ask her if I could use some of her insulin in the interim. He would be able to provide me with a replacement syringe and issue me with a prescription to take to the nearest chemist.

Resuming my story, as the nearest chemist was located in either Dingwell or Inverness, provided she had sufficient stocks for her own use, then I should ask this lady if she could let me have a 10cc vial of insulin or at least enough for me to use the following morning. However I must be sure to get to a chemist the next day.

The G.P. duly gave the trainee nurse directions to the farm and sent us on our way. The trip out to the farm really tested the car's springs and suspension and more than once its floor pan as the wheels desperately fought for traction on a wet mud and dung strewn track that had been deeply rutted by tractor wheels and was also dotted with frequent projections of the underlying granite substrata. However we eventually pulled up in the yard of a small farm holding to be greeted by a young woman whom I would estimate was in her late thirties. She ushered us into the house having been forewarned of our arrival by the G.P. who had advised her of the reason for our visit. She immediately engaged me in conversation about our shared condition and then, having ascertained that I needed to inject in the near future, insisted we stay and share tea with her and her husband which would be ready about an hour later and my companion readily agreed to this suggestion.

On further speaking to this young woman she confessed to me that she found it difficult to inject herself and had recently acquired a piece of apparatus which made the process a little easier. She then asked me if I would like to see it which I agreed that I would. I was intrigued that this clearly sensible and

---

individually responsible for managing and maintaining the condition themselves. Medics should only take over in emergency situations and take, in effect, a back seat offering advice and information only as and when requested by the patient, listening but not adopting a dictatorial role.

Before I resume my story I would urge any parent who may be reading this with a young diabetic themselves, to encourage their child / children to administer their own injections. The earlier they learn to do this the better and with the advent of insulin pens, which are far easier to use than syringes, they will soon become confident and proficient in the technique. It is inevitable they will need to do so for the rest of their lives. For the past sixty years there has been talk of breakthroughs in treatment. Essentially, however, with the possible exception of the insulin pump which has if, one is able to use it successfully, the understanding carbohydrate control, nothing has changed significantly since 1922 when Banting and Best discovered insulin. In nearly one hundred years, I would contend that the only real beneficiaries have been the drug companies. Diabetes has changed from a chronic medical condition to a highly profitable industry.

capable woman living in a very isolated location found it difficult to perform a task that was essential for the maintenance of her life.

She went to a Welsh dresser extracting a box about the size of a medium thickness paperback book from one of its drawers. She opened this to reveal what to me looked very similar to the skeleton of a pistol. She explained that once the syringe had been loaded with the required dosage it was then placed, complete with needle, on a carriage located at the top of the pistol-like object with the end of the syringe plunger placed against a shaped stop. There was a notched "V" at the opposite end of the carriage which had to be placed against the part of her body she was injecting. When the trigger was pulled the syringe would project forward so that the needle penetrated the skin to the required depth so delivering the syringe's contents. The whole mechanism was constructed from stainless steel and I could clearly see how this ingenious invention benefitted our kind host whom I suspected had at least a degree of needle phobia. However I declined her offer to try it on myself. I believe this was one of the best examples of innovative technology I have ever seen for the use of people like our host, who for whatever reason find it difficult to inject themselves. When I think this device was available as far back as 1957 I question the progress of today that Type One diabetics are constantly assured has been made!

Following a very pleasant meal with our host and her husband she gave me a 10cc vial of insulin from which we had both in turn drawn our respective evening requirements. This left about 2ccs remaining which she kindly insisted that I take away with me as she had a further vial available for herself. She then gave me the name and address of a chemist in Inverness which she used and was confident they would be able to fill the prescription which the G.P. had given to me earlier. We all then engaged in further conversation for a while and then after duly thanking this very kind lady for her help and wishing both her and her husband a pleasant goodbye myself and my companion took our leave and returned to the hostel.

This episode was then, and indeed remains so today, a prime example of how we all, each and everyone of us, are reliant on the preparedness of our fellow human beings to offer assistance to each other when the need is there. Indeed it is our moral duty to do so when we are in a position to offer such help and assistance and not in a manner that is either patronising or paternal. I wholeheartedly believe that society, whilst owing us all the chance to reach our full potential, should not prevent us from losing site of the fact that we in turn owe it to society to use that potential. We should not use it in order to gain personal wealth or aggrandisement but to use that potential for the benefit of society as a whole and of which we are all a part, irrespective of race, creed colour or nationality. The old adage of "do unto others as you would have them do unto you" is a concept well worth following.

The next morning Alan and I made our way into Inverness where we made the necessary visit to the chemist. Whilst there I discovered to my surprise that the thoughtful G.P. whom I had seen the day before, had also given me a prescription for a Bakelite case in which to contain my syringe as well as the insulin.

Leaving these premises Alan and I proceeded to explore the beautiful capital city of these highlands and eventually made it down to Edinburgh without further incident. Here we agreed to split up with Alan making his way down to Yorkshire to explore what little he knew for sure of his background prior to moving to London and myself proceeding to Middlesbrough on Teeside to renew an acquaintanceship I had previously had with another apprentice I had met at Esher who shared similar political beliefs.

Some weeks before this at a branch meeting one night which I had been Chairing the question had arisen as to the branch's nomination of a candidate for the forthcoming General Election. We had been supplied with a list of candidates by the local Walworth branch of the Labour Party, to which we were affiliated, and invited to make our selection. Accordingly each candidate had been invited to attend and asked in turn to address the branch. The last of these was a Ray Gunter who was the then General Secretary, or President, of the train drivers' union A.S.L.E.F. (Associated Society of Locomotive Engineers and Firemen). At the end of his address I could clearly see that the branch members had not been particularly impressed with his presentation so to save him embarrassment, as there was a notable lack of questions from the floor, I asked his opinion on a number of current issues including the past debacle at Suez. As I had anticipated this unnerved him somewhat.

I then asked him to explain his views on the Anglo-American alliance, the Cold War and the nuclear threat and after some fifteen minutes of incoherent rambling he completely destroyed what little chance he may have had of securing the nomination from the London Central No.2 E.T.U. branch. Before he left he suddenly turned to me and in a very indignant and patronising manner told me that I had a lot to learn about politics which was not all about being a revolutionary youngster. There followed an audible gasp of surprise from the thirty or so members present and he left the meeting with a crestfallen look on his face. This bitter retort must have been due to the realisation that he had definitely blown his chance of securing the branch's nomination. He did, however, go on to win Southwark in the General Election and subsequently served in Harold Wilson's cabinet but, to the best of my knowledge, he was never again invited to attend another E.T.U. branch meeting.

Joan

To return to the question of adding the Streatham Locarno to our list of dance venues, I can remember, one Saturday night in September 1957, having to catch a couple of buses, I made my way to Streatham where I expected to meet up with my two friends who had both agreed to make the Locarno our destination that weekend. When I arrived, around 7.00 p.m., which was our customary meeting time, I was surprised to see a queue some three hundred yards long and at least the width of four or five people, spreading across the whole width of the pavement. Knowing the doors were due to open at 7.15 p.m. I knew the queue would not take long to disperse so I slowly made my way to the rear hoping to catch sight of one or other of my friends. However this proved not to be the case for the youths gathered there came from all over the south east and south west of London and the queue must have contained in the region of eight hundred people, there being not one face amongst them I could recognise.

On reaching the end of the queue I duly took my place in line assuming my friends had been delayed. Amongst the young men in the queue there was a preponderance of, what at that time, was known as the Edwardian or "Teddy boy" suits. These were three buttoned single breasted suits, usually charcoal grey in colour, with a black velvet collar and worn with a white double cuffed shirt and black string tie. The girls accompanying these lads would be wearing pencil skirts sometimes with a coat similar to their male partners but more often with a white or grey blouse and a waistcoat and stiletto shoes.

There could also be seen signs of the newly emerging Italian style, or full drape style, jacket which was beginning to find favour. The main difference between these various modes of dress, as far as the young lads were concerned, was the trousers that the Teddy boys wore as opposed to the Italian style, more usually known as drainpipe. They had no turnups at the bottom and were fourteen inches in width. The drape jacket hung at least two inches or more below the hip and would be worn with trousers that did have turnups and were eighteen inches at the base. They were invariably worn with thick crepe soled shoes known as "brothel creepers".

Most of the girls who wore dresses followed the so-called "A" line style which had been introduced in Paris over the last couple of years. Most, however, chose to wear skirts and blouses in a range of colours although green seemed to be a frequent favourite.

When I started to go dancing, much to the amusement of my closest friends but with the encouragement of my parents, my mother and Colleen in particular, I had bought a semi drape, single breasted link button grey suit and drainpipe trousers made to measure which I wore only for visits to dance halls. I had purchased this dance attire at the Burtons clothes store which was then known as the "fifty bob tailor". At all other times I tended to wear blue jeans and a drill type shirt, i.e. two breast pockets.

My uncle Bert, who had a large collection of ties, looked in disdain at the so-called "slim Jim" tie I had bought to wear with my dance rig and passed on to me a number of his own ties spending thirty minutes teaching me the knack of tying the Windsor knot. The whole outfit was completed by the purchase of a pair of black mock crocodile, pointed toe, Italian style shoes which were so soft and flexible that by bending the sole the toe could be bought right round to fit inside the heel. I have never since possessed a pair of shoes that were as comfortable as those.

So, dressed in my dance rig I waited at the Locarno all the while scanning the youths joining up behind me on watch for my friends' arrival. I inevitably reached the front which presented me with a real dilemma; with neither of them having arrived I did not know if I should continue inside or not. The girls already inside, if not dancing with a male partner would invariably be dancing in pairs so without another male to accompany me I could see no chance of splitting up and pairing off with a couple of girls. With the pressure mounting behind me I was forced to make a decision. I could either go inside and hope there was another lone male like myself or give up and return home so saving on the admission price, which was not an insignificant sum to a nineteen year old apprentice. It would, however, also mean bearing the cost of a wasted bus fare. I had not inherited my father's gambling instincts but on this occasion I decided to make an exception so I paid up and went inside.

By this time the dance hall was quite full with many young men standing around the periphery of the dance floor and a few of them dancing, presumably with the girls they had entered with. The majority of the girls were on the dance floor in pairs with only a few standing around. I looked around in vain for a male in the same position as myself but after some twenty fruitless minutes I gave up on that endeavour the main reason being that during my constant scan of the dance hall my attention had continually been drawn to a tall slim brunette who was dancing with a blond girl a good thirty centimetres shorter than herself. I stood at 1.87 metres tall and estimated that the brunette girl was perhaps some 50 millimetres shorter than myself and she was not wearing stilettos. She was therefore quite a tall girl, head and shoulders above the average. What is more she had beautiful lustrous dark hair which hung almost to the small of her back. She exactly matched up to what had always been my ideal.

Taking one final desperate look around for another single male but without any success I knew I had to face up to the possibility of being rejected. Nevertheless I also knew that I would always regret it if I did not try so I nervously and awkwardly threaded my way through the throng of dancers until I reached my goal. Finally standing beside the girl I had had my eye on I tentatively asked if I might have the next dance apologising for the fact that I was alone. In some surprise, I assumed at my audacity, she turned to her blond friend who, with a glance at her blushing brunette partner and a mocking smile said, "go ahead, but with his height he probably has big feet so watch your toes". With that the blond girl turned and walked off the dance floor leaving me to dance with the pretty brunette. I was somewhat disconcerted to discover that she was a far more proficient dancer than I had anticipated and in fact the warning of her blond friend proved to work in reverse! However we managed a couple of quick steps without too much of a problem but, for me, the foxtrot was way beyond my capability so, at her suggestion, we simply bobbed from side to side whilst we exchanged names and a few brief details. Coincidently it turned out that both she and her blond friend had the same name which was Joan.

As the band left the stage for a break they were replaced by a D.J. with a batch of rock and roll records. Joan and I made our way off the dance floor to locate her friend of the same name who once found, to my surprise, indicated that it would be OK for us to return to the dance floor. In order to bring as many people onto the dance floor as possible before starting the rock and roll session the D.J. indicated that he intended to firstly play a slow number that was rapidly climbing the music charts at that time. So to the strains of Nat King Cole's "When I Fall in Love" Joan and I returned to the dance floor.

A little later we noticed that her friend had also been asked to dance so with clear consciences we danced together for the remainder of the session. It subsequently emerged that the two Joans had met some two months previously when they had both started working for the British American Tobacco Company and were undergoing training prior to being assigned to respective clerical posts. Since their initial meeting they had spent alternate weekends at each other's homes staying over and then setting off to work together on the Monday morning.

The evening I met "my" Joan, her blond friend was staying with her that evening at her home in Vauxhall, planning to return to her own home in

Bromley the next morning, Sunday. I established this information on the bus that all three of us boarded to take us from Streatham to Vauxhall from where there was a direct route to where I lived in Peckham. I offered to walk them home as their route was pretty dark and took them through a series of back streets. It also meant passing a number of notorious pubs where, after closing time, groups of people would usually be standing outside to continue their night's drinking after purchasing bottles at "last orders".

When we reached the block of flats where "my" Joan lived, on the fourth floor, not wishing to climb the stairs I asked her if we could perhaps meet the following night to go to the pictures. After checking with her blond friend that she was still intending to return home the next day she agreed and suggested we meet at 7.00 p.m. at the entrance to the Oval underground station which would be more convenient for both of us. This venue was both well lit and the closest to the cinema at the Elephant & Castle, which I had nominated, and she could walk there with no concern. This being arranged I took my leave and hurried off to catch the last number thirty six bus to Peckham.

The following evening I duly arrived at the Oval tube station ten minutes before our appointed meeting time. At about ten minutes past seven I noticed a group of people standing at the bus stop on the opposite side of the road so I made my way across to check whether Joan was amongst them. Seeing that she was not I started to suspect that she may have stood me up and broken our date.

However I decided I would walk to the corner to check along the route we had followed the previous evening and through the steady drizzle that was falling from an overcast sky I saw a figure come into view wearing a long swagger coat the upturned collar of which hid any view of either the face or the hair. The height of the figure approaching suggested this may perhaps be my date. As I had often been told, I myself was usually quite recognisable from a distance due to my rolling gait. Given my limited knowledge of the fairer sex at that time the figure coming towards me could have been either sex. This uncertainty turned to confirmation that the approaching figure was indeed the Joan I had met the night previously but on reaching the corner where I was waiting she walked straight past me heading for the bus stop.

Utterly devastated I remained where I was for a while longer and then in some despair decided I should at least try to ascertain if the mistake was on my part so I walked back to the bus stop. Approaching her and in some trepidation, I said "excuse me but are we not supposed to be going to the pictures together?" Following a moment's hesitation she moved aside her collar which she had been clenching tightly round her face. Upon seeing me standing there her face initially lost its colour then, as recognition dawned, flushed in deep embarrassment. A series of sincere but abject apologies followed until I, now myself very embarrassed, held up my hand palm upwards and in a mock Yiddish accent said "enough already, enough". The ice broken we both broke into fits of unrestrained laughter.

Over the years this episode was to raise many a laugh and expressions of disbelief from amongst our friends and Joan's female acquaintances. She would take great delight in relating the tale of how she very nearly managed to avoid the relationship which, from that initial near miss, was to develop, blossom and endure for just a few weeks short of fifty years.

We rapidly crossed the road to where we had been due to meet and descended to the platform for the short journey to the Trocadero Cinema at the Elephant & Castle where we hoped to be in time to catch the start of the film, Oklahoma, which Joan had told me her mother had seen on stage.

The reason for our earlier mishap was cleared up at the start of the film when Joan reached into her handbag to withdraw a pair of glasses which she then put on and I realised she had been unable to see me clearly. I grinningly reassured her that the old adage that men do not make passes at girls who wore glasses was absolute rubbish and proceeded to reach into the breast pocket of my suit, which I had worn again to hopefully make a favourable impression, and donned my own pair of glasses. These had been acquired some weeks previously after enduring months of headaches which finally forced me to visit an optician. There it had been confirmed that although I was not short sighted my vision was biased more towards near rather than distant objects which the glasses I had been prescribed evened out.

Joan's situation was the reverse of mine but on our first date we had both made the same error of not wearing our glasses to create an impression and with the added element of the drizzling rain had failed to identify each other for sure following or brief encounter of the previous evening.

The film over we decided we would walk back to Vauxhall which was some two miles distant. This would give us an opportunity to talk and get to know each other better. I did enquire of her if she realised just how far it was but she rather disdainfully rejected the implied suggestion that she would perhaps find it easier to take the bus. She insisted that walking would give us an opportunity to learn more about each other's backgrounds, families, likes and dislikes, etc. I very soon realised that Joan was an intelligent, serious and sincere individual and I hoped I would be able to make an intense favourable impression on her as she was rapidly making upon me.

In the time it took for us to walk home I discovered that Joan, or Jo as I was later to call her, was a true Cockney, having been born in Bow hospital in January 1940. She had spent the war years in New Herrington in Durham at the home of her grandparents and her grandfather had been a miner. Her father had been a fusilier in the Royal Inniskilling Fusiliers and had served with the 8th Army from Alamein through the Sicilian and Italian campaigns and had been demobbed in 1946. On his return the family had been reunited and lived in rented rooms at Kings Cross until they had been allocated a London County Council flat in Vauxhall.

Joan had left school as a seventeen year old two months previously having been Head Girl at Vauxhall Grammar School. She had, for a time, been in the Guides and had also taught youngsters at Sunday School. Furthermore she had recently returned from a holiday in Belgium which she had undertaken together with one of her school friends. She told me that she corresponded with a young man named George who was serving in the navy as a conscript but he was a penfriend rather than a boyfriend.

Joan had no siblings but did have two male cousins who lived in Durham the eldest of whom, Alec, she regarded as the closest thing to an elder brother she had. He was six months older than herself and a year younger than me. She told me that Alec was an apprentice shipwright in a yard in Sunderland and was later to become a highly qualified ships engineer who was held in deep regard by his colleagues.

Other than initial amazement that I needed to inject myself twice daily to stay healthy, Joan did not seem at all disconcerted about the details I revealed about my own background, including my affiliation to the Y.C.L. and agnosticism. So, after a kiss goodnight and arrangements to meet again later that week, as I headed for the bus stop to go home I can remember telling myself that I did not think this would be a brief teenage relationship. Joan was a very intelligent working class girl whose opinions and observations on matters such as atomic weapons, apartheid, health and housing had made a big impression on me during our conversations on that first walk home, yet she was still only seventeen and a half years old. Our only disagreement had been her rating Frankie Vaughan's talent as a singer which I could not agree with.

Over the course of the next few months we grew even closer but I was still somewhat surprised when, in early March 1958, she announced her intention to join me on the section of that year's Aldermaston march coming through East London to meet the West London contingent in Trafalgar Square. So, together with myself, Joan and Alan joined the march at Gardiner's Corner in Stepney. As usual during Easter in London it was raining steadily and slightly chilly. Joan was wearing a light mackintosh over a dress and cardigan as was

Alan whilst I wore my ex-R.A.F. duffle coat. By the time we reached the building in Fenchurch Street where a couple of weeks previously I had been within seconds of being electrocuted, Joan was soaked to the skin. In the basement of the firm's lock-up I knew there were a number of donkey jackets so I figured if I could just gain access then I could get one for her.

The fact that the building was now occupied was due to the reason I had nearly lost my life. Arrangements had been made to isolate the electrical supply to the upper floors. I had removed the cover to the rising main on the thirteenth floor and was reaching into it to disconnect the necessary cables from the bus bars when the bell indicating the lift had reached the thirteenth floor could be heard. This should have been impossible as the rising main was supposedly dead. The lift doors opened and a voice screamed at me to stop in a clearly worried tone. This turned out to be the foreman who explained that the arrangement to isolate the electrical supply had been overridden by some commercial clown who had instructed their maintenance staff to switch the supply back on and they, in their non-technical ignorance, had done so. Just when the lift bell had rung I had been on the point of receiving a 440v to earth which would have meant certain death.

Anyway handing Joan my duffle coat I managed, after some effort, to rouse the building's new commissionaire and explained to him the problem with her wet mac, which was now draped over my arm, and my intention to get one of the donkey jackets that were stored in the lock-up; she was also in need of the toilet. Despite his protestations however my unremitting pressure finally achieved my objective and with Joan now fully protected inside the jacket I had procured we proceeded to join the 100,000 other marchers now gathered in Trafalgar Square. We arrived just in time to hear Aneurin Bevan, or Nye as he was known, give his address. As we made our way home that day I knew deep inside that I had met my soulmate.

Two weeks later, after assessing Jo's ability on a push bike, it was obvious she would not be up to the task of cycling all the way to Brighton for the day so we decided to take the train. We spent an enjoyable day skimming pebbles picked up from the hoards scattered across the beach, walking along the pier and round the outside of the Pavilion. As a staunch republican my loathing of all things regal kept me outside of this building but Jo made no objection to this; she too harboured anti monarchical thoughts.

As evening started to draw in we decided to get some fish and chips before catching the train home so walking back inland and up the High Street we entered a mews where a queue had formed outside a fish friers. I retrieved my syringe and insulin from out of Joan's handbag where I had put it to keep it safe and stepped inside a shop doorway to administer my usual injection. As I emerged two women of around fifty in age passed me muttering their disgust to each other at such action, wrongly assuming I was taking drugs.

I rejoined Jo just as she entered the shop and placed our order where I stood next to her at the counter. I again placed my syringe and insulin into her bag for safe keeping. I paid for our order which was handed to Jo and we turned to leave the shop. As we emerged, however, a hand was placed on my shoulder and I was propelled firmly forward with the words "your are under arrest"! Upon turning and much to my surprise I was confronted with a policeman. I asked him what I was supposed to have done and was informed that I had been seen supposedly "shooting" drugs. I was then frog-marched down the mews and placed into the back of a waiting patrol car. Jo, meanwhile, was hurrying down the mews after me shouting "let him go, he's diabetic". When she reached the patrol car she frantically banged on the roof till the policeman on the passenger side wound down the window. She insisted that I be allowed to eat my meal warning that I could be dead in half an hour if I did not eat something. Their only response was to invite her to accompany me to the station.

So together we arrived at the police station where I was required to empty my pockets and then go down to the cells. As I was being led down, above Joan's frantic protests, I heard the desk sergeant on the telephone requesting the attendance of a police doctor. About ten minutes later, now some twenty five minutes after I had injected the insulin, the cell door opened and a man entered. He took one look at me and ordered the police officer who had opened the door to quickly get me a cup of tea with plenty of sugar. I was by now sweating quite profusely and the man, whom I presumed was the doctor, asked me how much insulin I had taken and why had I not taken any glucose. I responded that I had had sixteen units and that the desk sergeant had taken my glucose off of me.

The tea arrived and the doctor ordered me to drink it as quickly as I could. He then asked me who my Consultant was and I replied that it was Dr Lawrence. He said "in that case you do not need me to tell you to drink the tea quickly". He went on to say that I had obviously explained my condition to my girlfriend and that I had quite some girl there. She had been giving the desk sergeant a real ear bashing! As I put the cup down the doctor turned towards the door beckoning for me to follow. When we got to the desk the sergeant was instructed to get the fish and chips re-heated and after we had eaten them he was to organise transport to the rail station.

My belongings were returned to me and the sergeant and doctor went off into an office. Joan and I had finished our meal by the time the sergeant re-emerged and a police driver was instructed to take us to the station and to make sure we caught our train safely. We were also told never to return to Brighton.

So, safely ensconced on the train, I turned to Joan determined I was not going to lose this girl, and asked her to marry me. I told her not to reply immediately but to take time to think about it. I told her I loved her, not just because of the afternoon's events but all I had seen and learned of her actions and attitudes over the past six months. Jo gave me her answer when we met on the following Wednesday evening. Forty nine years later I learned that her mother, Isobel, had advised her to think long and hard about my proposal because with my condition I would always be unwell. Isobel herself had suffered a nervous breakdown which I believe she felt was caused as a result of the Post Traumatic Stress Disorder (PTSD) that her husband, Albert, suffered with following the war.

However, fortunately for me, Jo rejected her mother's advice telling her that she was not bothered about my condition and that she loved me. I had no inkling of this conversation between mother and daughter when I met up with Jo that following Wednesday evening. To my intense joy and delight she kissed me and said yes to my proposal. However she said that we now had a problem and when I asked her what that was she replied that none of the girls she worked with would believe she was engaged in the absence of a ring. Grinning happily I conceded that in order to rectify this we should go window shopping. So on that Saturday afternoon we went off into town to buy a ring and make it formal.

When I relayed my good news to my parents they were delighted having taken an immediate liking to Joan after I had invited her for Sunday dinner about a month or so after we had first met. Similarly, from what I could tell, Jo's parents reciprocated this feeling towards myself.

With my twentieth birthday rapidly approaching we decided to make a day of it and lunch at Freddie Mills, a newly opened Chinese restaurant. When we had finished our meal Joan jokingly told me that she wanted a proper marriage proposal from me. So, in a restaurant full of people, I duly went down on one knee in front of her and formally proposed. With a brief moment of hesitation, for dramatic effect, she accepted. This brought an immediate round of applause from the other diners who all wished us both luck for the future. One even went so far as to buy a bottle of wine in order to offer up a toast. Deliriously happy and with Jo wearing her brand new engagement ring, we left the restaurant with the good wishes of all inside ringing in our ears. We went on from there to the Astoria in Tottenham Court Road where we watched the film "South Pacific". Now, looking back, some fifty one years on, that was certainly a very special and enchanted afternoon.

From the start we both decided to save hard in order to give us a good start in setting up a home with furniture, household equipment, etc., without the weight of debt hanging round our necks. We unanimously decided that we would like to have two children and that Joan would give up work when our first child came along.

So far as accommodation was concerned, given the acute housing shortage resulting from wartime losses and population increase, whilst we realised that we stood very little chance of securing any Local Authority housing we did, however, register with our respective Boroughs. An ancillary advantage of doing this was that this would automatically place us on the so-called industrial housing scheme which, in the event of you being able to secure employment in an area where your particular skills were required, then accommodation would be made available to you by the Local Authority in that area.

All these hopes and dreams were made during our now regular evening strolls from Vauxhall when, at some point in our walk, we would usually sit down on a bench in St James' Park, about thirty metres back from the water's edge. Even before we had had the opportunity of sharing a kiss or lighting a cigarette the ducks and geese on the lake would start quacking and squawking which became a constant source of amusement to us and invariably reduced Joan into helpless fits of laughter. The number of times we were actually able to beat the birds in this endeavour in the eighteen months or so of the duration of our engagement were probably no more than can be counted on one hand.

The time was by now fast approaching when I was due to sit the final examination for my City & Guilds certification. Most of the commercial and retail work undertaken by my employers was carried out in outlets in Curzon and Bond Streets with the majority of the domestic work on premises in Hampstead and Chelsea. For the past six months I had been one out of the star pair the firm employed there and I was confident I could pass the examination. I decided to approach the firm's Managing Director with a proposal that I spend some time in the drawing office. This request was initially met with some deliberation but he could obviously tell that I was really determined. He resorted to trying to bargain with me saying that if I did indeed achieve the City & Guilds certification then I would be the first one to do so in which case he would consider it. I did achieve a second degree pass so approached the Managing Director again who, although reluctant, did agree this time.

A few weeks later I was approached by one of the Contracts Managers, as their so-called engineers were known, who enquired if I could work out a lighting scheme. I assured him that provided I was supplied with the relevant detail of the area in question, including the use to which it was to be put, i.e. nature of activity proposed, then I felt sure that I could come up with a feasible design.

The next day he gave me a roll of drawings for a three floor building which would be occupied by the Cherry Blossom Polish Company. A few days later I handed the drawings back to him having worked out the different luminosity intensity details and the number of lighting points required on each floor that would be required for the different activities envisaged. He was clearly very impressed with the detail I had gone into and announced his intention to submit the drawings to the company for inclusion with the tenders they would be making for the installation contract.

He was back again by the end of the week and returned the drawings to me telling me they had now been issued to the ten major installation firms in London with the company's tender for the work on that building. He put it to me that as I had made such a good job of the drawings would I be interested in drawing up the tender. This made me question what he was employed for but unable to refuse a challenge I agreed to try. Accordingly I spent the next week or so working out circuitry, phase balancing, diversity, cable sizes, conduit capacities, labour requirement, etc., knowing full well that price rings and fixing was rampant in the electrical contracting industry.

Using the practical experience I had gained in the four years I had been working, I tried my utmost to be accurate but also fair to my colleagues who would be responsible for the work with regard to the time allocated for the completion of the installation. I was pleasantly surprised when some two weeks later, to the astonishment of everyone in the Drawing Office, the Contracts Manager congratulated and informed me that the tender had been successful and Berkeley Electricals had been awarded the contract.

The Contracts Manager then told me the Managing Director wanted to see me and on entering his office I got the impression that he was in a far more outgoing and pleasant mood than I had seen him in on any of our other previous encounters. He motioned for me to sit down and asked if I had given any thought to what I planned to do in the next two months and after that upon the completion of my apprenticeship. I responded that I intended to earn as much money as possible for I was getting married in October. He asked me if I would consider accepting a post as Junior Engineer emphasising the normal middle class promise of a glittering career, promotion, etc. He said that in his long experience, I had already proven to be the most competent apprentice he had ever come across.

My first question was to ask what the wage would be for this position, followed by a request for his explanation as to why he had shown such initial reluctance to allow me to work in the Drawing Office. He took some time to respond to this, all the while seemingly examining the top of his desk and also the ceiling in some detail. He finally told me that some two years previous he had been approached by Special Branch who had informed him that I had been distributing subversive literature at the Borough Polytechnic and as a result I was now someone they were monitoring. Furthermore, aware of my involvement with the union, he had been suspicious of my motives. However, he now had to admit that he had been wrong and therefore wanted me to accept the proffered post which would initially be paid at the skilled rate.

I was astounded that a mere eighteen year old merited the attention of Special Branch. I responded that in order for me to build up the confidence I felt was necessary to be responsible for a mate as well as myself I would consequently like to return to the tools until I finished my time. He reluctantly accepted this telling me he had never met anyone less in need of self confidence than myself.

I later relayed the details of this meeting to my father who said that when I had finished my time I would need to build up a bit of a reputation as a good and competent spark pretty quickly because it was pretty obvious I was potentially on the way to being blacklisted. After imparting this warning and sound advice my father, with a delighted grin, said "you certainly appear to have given that smug bastard the lesson he deserved and being successful in winning that tender sets you well on the way to proving your competence".

He then asked me what Joan's reaction had been which I felt was an interesting question. Since I had told her about the offer she had repeatedly asked me if I was making the right decision to which I had responded that I most definitely had. She then went on to say to me "now I am going to put those toffee nosed snobs at the office in their place". Eighteen months previously Joan had successfully completed her initial assessment and been appointed as an Account Clerk in the Shareholder Account Office. During her time there she had made quite an impression on her colleagues demonstrating both her intelligence and ability. When she had informed them that we were getting engaged they had expressed disappointment believing she deserved something much better than a "oike"[3] who worked on a building site.

---

3   Middle class slang dating from the early 1900s

During the two weeks remaining of my apprenticeship I gave a lot of thought to the question of taking on the responsibility as lead member of a pair. I finally decided to remove myself from the environment of the contracting industry and made an approach to London County Council seeking a position with them. This secured I was told to report with my tools to their depot at the fire station in Whitechapel. Over the past four years I had been gradually assembling my electrician's tool kit which, in the early 1960s, consisted entirely of hand tools. However, at that time, with the possible exception of brick laying, an electrician had, of necessity, to also have a basic knowledge and a degree of proficiency in carpentry, plastering, etc., and his tool kit had to reflect this. The whole kit would weigh in the region of fifty six pounds and had to be carried by hand around and between the confines of sites with mud, scaffolding, ladders, etc., all needing to be negotiated. However this rarely gave me any problems where my diabetes was concerned.

The task assigned to me on that first day was to sort out a recurring problem with the lighting in a local school and the mate assigned to me was a man of about my father's age. On our way to the site he warned me I would need to watch myself and be careful. Intrigued, I asked why. The only response he would give me was "you will find out".

We arrived on site which I expected to be a junior school but to my horror I discovered it was actually an all female senior school with nearly one thousand, fifteen and sixteen year old pupils. I immediately understood and appreciated my mate's warning.

We were able to quickly establish that the fault was entirely due to the deterioration of the VIR cables with which the school was wired. These were not only problematic but extremely dangerous so I recommended that a complete re-wire was needed. This same problem had been the cause of the fire we had witnessed in 1954 which had spread through the roof of the school in Adey's Road.

We were subsequently given the go ahead to carry out this work and following my mate's advice turned up the following day wearing jeans rather than the cord shorts I had worn the previous day. He had been worried that I would set a precedent that others would find it difficult to match. The school's Head Mistress had also drawn attention to my "inappropriate" dress code.

The complete re-wiring of that school was finished in three weeks and I could not get out of there fast enough. As a slim six foot twenty one year old I found that every time I climbed just two steps up the ladder there would be titters and giggles from a host of nubile young girls. Unfortunately our work had to be done during the school day when it was fully occupied and functioning. Joan thought my discomfiture at this scenario was hilarious. Thankfully I never had to repeat this experience, nor did I want to!

Over the eighteen months between finishing my apprenticeship and getting married I changed employers almost as often as I changed socks working in exhibition halls such as The Furniture - Ideal Homes - Wedding and another name which now escapes me. The sparks employed to these names were supplied via the Area Office and as I thought I had had my share of the big money they paid compared to contracting rates, I subsequently quit and found a job with a small firm where most of their work was carried out in the West End.

The first job I undertook was at the Palladium Theatre and upon arrival waited there for the mate who was to work with me at that venue. When he arrived he seemed somewhat nervous so I suggested we retire to a nearby café for a cup of tea which would give us the chance to get to know each other. As we sat down he said he hoped that I would not object to his paper and nervously reached into his jacket pocket. I similarly reached into my own jacket pocket and withdrew my own paper. His face suddenly beamed as he realised that we both read the same newspaper – The Daily Worker. He introduced himself and for some reason which I felt was completely unnecessary told me that he was a Jew. His name was Gerry Gable, an aspiring journalist/novelist who had been advised to try his luck as an electrician's mate so that he could earn enough money to support his ambitions. We became firm friends and worked together for the next six months or so for various different firms. Gerry subsequently went on to publish the anti fascist magazine "Searchlight".

Following the period working for exhibitions my name also came to the top of the area list for the film studios where I was fortunate enough to work on the gantry of one of the major hits at that time. I spent eight hours a day some thirty feet above the floor in pitch black darkness working on a twenty four inch gantry where I had to occasionally strike one of the three 3kw arc lights and apply the necessary shrouds in order to direct the beam. This was boring in the extreme, the only compensation being the pay which was the best available outside the print[4] in the London area. The subject onto whom the spotlight was directed was either Graham Stark, Peter Sellers or, most impressively, Sophia Loren, for the film being shot was "The Millionairess". There were few greater pleasures for a young male than controlling a spotlight on a sight as beautiful as women like Sophia Loren who, now in her mid 70s, still looks great today.

After the completion of that film and another "B" movie, the long hours of

---

4   Newspapers & Publishing, i.e. Odhams Press

inactivity and the journey out to Borehamwood, Pinewood or Elstree, started to get on my nerves so I returned to contracting. Gerry and I worked as a pair for various firms and whilst working on a site one day we found a discarded bowler hat and a top hat. Henceforth, when off site at either our tea or dinner breaks, we could be found wearing them and doffing them at any passing attractive female which caused great amusement to all concerned. Much to our amusement, when working in the City, we would similarly doff our hats to any so-called "city gent", much to their consternation and annoyance.

One such memorable occasion, having rigged a halo from a piece of draught proofing tape, we went down to the Lost Property Office in Selfridges and Gerry said to the man behind the counter "excuse me but I appear to have lost my harp, has it perchance been handed in?" this said with a deadpan expression. People in the area looked bemused, some with a slight smile on their faces and others quite perplexed. I stood hatless a few feet back seemingly the next customer. The man turned shaking his head and said "he has certainly lost something but it is not his bloody harp" and with that he beat a hasty retreat before anyone else could approach the counter. Such little amusements served to lighten the pressure of our working environment.

At around this time my great aunt had enquired of her landlord if he was aware of any vacant accommodation as her nephew was looking for a flat. As a result, some months later Joan and I were invited to attend for an interview with him at his house in Ealing in West London. This interview proved to be far more in-depth and intrusive in its detail than any similar experience I had had when seeking employment. However it did eventually lead to the offer of a ground floor flat in a dilapidated condition situated in Clapham. If we accepted, it would be our responsibility to bring it up to habitable standard.

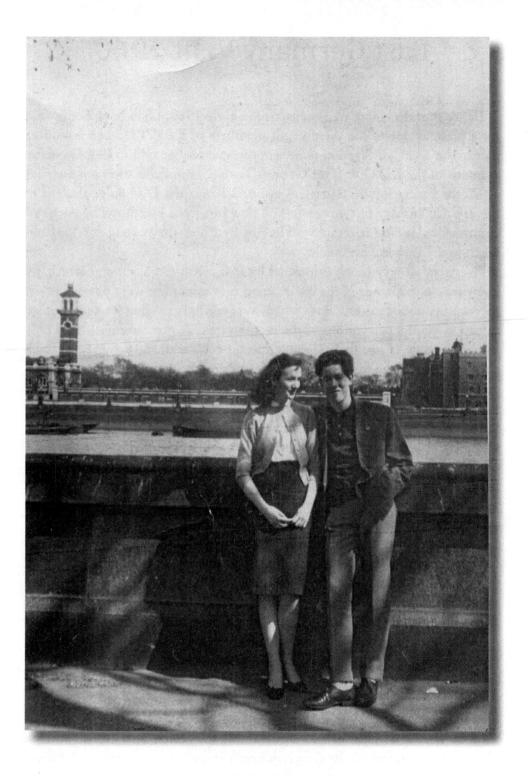

October 1958, London on the Embankment

East Germany Visit 1960

Three months before we got married in early 1960, I had been nominated for a place as one of the three youth members of the E.T.U. who would be part of the T.U.C. delegation to be sent on an exchange visit to East Germany as guests of the F.D.G.B. (Free German Trade Union Federation – a member of World Federation of Trade Unions) which was the D.D.R. equivalent to the T.U.C. In May of that year we all flew out from Heathrow by Airspeed Ambassador landing at Templehoff in East Berlin where we were collected and taken to a T.U. hotel for lunch.

We were all very much impressed by that swish establishment which we knew was in the hands of the trade union movement but were puzzled at the incongruity of our surroundings which were contrary to what we had been led to expect via the perceptions of the western media's presentations. As I only knew the name of one truly German meal, i.e. eisbahn and sauerkraut which although not on the menu, I decided I would order that so I went ahead and ordered pork and pickled cabbage. However I received my comeuppance when it eventually arrived on a plate the size of a tray! The joint of pork was at least the size of my head and the cabbage, I am sure, would have filled a small bucket. I protested that a meal that size would be enough to feed a family of four back home and I only required a normal German worker's meal. I was assured that Germans were big meat eaters and was now faced with, quite literally, a very large problem. The meal in front of me contained no carbohydrates without which my blood sugar level would collapse yet if I ate the meal how on earth would I be able to find room in my stomach to further consume the essential carbohydrates? The answer soon presented itself for one of my colleagues had ordered gateaux for his sweet so I would do the same. Therefore, with abject apologies I managed to eat about sixty percent of the pork and perhaps thirty percent of the cabbage and then being unable to consume another mouthful gratefully accepted a proffered cigar and smoked that before eating a small piece of gateaux in order to meet my body's carbohydrate requirements.

The meal was delicious but none of us truly believed it in any way resembled what was normally eaten by a German worker in the same way that a meal at The Ritz would in no way resemble that eaten by a British worker. However, as our experiences over the next month were to prove, I believe that was the only occasion either consciously or unconsciously there was any attempt to mislead us regarding the position of the working class in the eastern sector, i.e. the D.D.R. (German Democratic Republic), in May 1960.

Two things on that trip particularly impressed me. In order to liaise and discuss matters of concern with our German counterparts we were taken to a trade union rest/holiday home in the Hartz Mountains where we spent out time in daily debates and discussions with our German colleagues. As the weather was exceedingly warm we asked if there was a swimming pool anywhere in the vicinity. Having been advised there was indeed one in a nearby village which may be open together with a young girl named Sue, a S.O.G.A.T. (Society of Graphical and Allied Trades) delegate, I set off that evening to locate it.

On reaching the village it looked to us to be deserted but as we passed what appeared to be a disused station we heard music emanating from inside so we opened a door and went in. On entering we found a gathering of about forty people listening to a group of musicians who were playing the accordion, violin and tuba. One man detached himself from the group of spectators and came over to us. Using what few words of German we knew, together with numerous hand and arm gestures, we endeavoured to communicate with him. Sue and I were each handed a stein (beer mug) and asked if we would be willing to talk to our host's twelve year old daughter who was learning to speak English and she would be very grateful for the practise. We readily agreed to this and asked if she had a textbook handy. To our amazement when she produced her textbook we found it contained a quite detailed story of an English family and their participation in and on the Aldermaston march. For a twelve year old, we discovered that the child's ability in English was far superior to what either myself or Sue had achieved at the same age in either the French or German we had been respectively taught. The content of her story was also much more in line with our common human desire for peace.

The other thing that impressed us was an exceedingly emotional visit to Buchenwald concentration camp. This camp dealt specifically with trade unionists, anti-fascists and left wing political prisoners. In the east we were assured that all children in their early teens visited this or other similar camps in order to learn about their country's past history under fascism. Accordingly, coinciding with our visit, we noted there were quite a number of school parties being taken round the site. It was also noted that not a single bird could be seen or heard and nature, in all its aspects, appeared to have entirely deserted the environment.

We also visited factory complexes in Magdeburg where, as guests of the Workers' Committee, we were able to examine the facilities and working conditions. By common agreement we all felt that in most cases these were superior to our own in comparable enterprises. There was one thing however which did not impress either myself or another of my E.T.U. colleagues. At one factory site we stood looking at the conduits carrying the cables into the top of the main switchboard distributing the electricity supply to the factory. The conduits entered the board at all sorts of angles and were what only could be described as one hell of a mess. We were used to installing conduits in a symmetrical manner so that all bends, sets and double sets ran parallel to each other to look aesthetically pleasing. This "cat's cradle approach, whilst achieving its purpose we felt was slap dash in the extreme.

We encountered a similar situation in Berlin when a number of us connected with the building trade had asked to be taken to a site at which I for one was initially impressed and not just because the site Works Committee were continually plying us with bottles of beer, although of course they were very acceptable.

It was claimed they were erecting three storey blocks of maisonettes in just one month from the ground to occupancy. The three of us who went on that visit considered this to be a great exaggeration and, in view of the grave housing shortage in the UK, asked how this was possible. On entering the site we had been puzzled by the presence of a large gantry crane on rails rather than the tower cranes with which we were familiar. Furthermore, on the periphery of the site, we could see large mounds of rubble with a piece of heavy equipment close by that was completely unknown to us. However the use of this piece of equipment was soon to become clear. Bulldozers and bucket lifts deposited the rubble into a hopper on top of a stone mill in which it was crushed. It was then mixed with concrete slurry and poured into moulds under the gantry rails. Twenty four hours later the slurry had set into preformed front, back, ends, roof, staircases and floors. The whole structure would then be lifted and transported by the gantry to an already prepared foundation plate where they would be assembled flat-pack style. The plumbing, electrics, door and window frames were also prepared in kit form. Each flat pack block was identical in construction and, in effect, mass produced.

Another thing about the site that surprised us was the scaffolding which was constructed of timber that was similar in diameter to the steel tubing type we were used to. We were informed that this timber scaffolding performed equally well but being somewhat sceptical a couple of us proceeded to hang, bounce and swing on it to test its strength. However we could discern no significant difference.

One further facet that a plumber colleague and myself raised was with regard to our respective trades. I could see no evidence of lighting switches. The only possible trace was about 200mm above the floor where a cable protruded from the wall at the approximate site of where we would place a power socket. Via our translator, whom I believe was somewhat hampered by the technical nature of our discussion, the General Foreman attempted to explain that the lighting switch was there for the children. I was struck by the apparent stupidity of his response so I further asked how a little old lady would manage to bend that far. In exasperation over his response the interpreter made some derogatory remark about the General Foreman in English and the plumber who was equally exasperated, together with myself, settled for another proffered beer.

We were by now approaching the end of our visit but we had two further surprises in store. The first occurred the following day when a number of our group had gone via the underground to West Berlin. Sue and I decided we would look at the shopping available in the east. I was particularly looking for an East European recording of the Jewish folk song "Havana Guila". When we had located a record store I was surprised to find a number of American servicemen, all in uniform, browsing among the records. They told me it was quite a common occurrence for many of them to come across the border to buy, as they put it, "hi brow" music. Their only difficulty in this regard was getting through "check point Charlie" on their side of the border. Unfortunately I had no luck with my own quest but I did purchase an L.P. of Romanian gypsy music. I also bought examples of German wood carving folk art for the family in the Hartz and an amber pendant for Joan.

That evening there was scheduled to be a public open air performance in Stalin Alley by Paul Robson which we were all looking forward to attending. He was in fine voice and we thoroughly enjoyed the performance together with the quarter million other people present on that memorable evening. I must, however, admit to not being very impressed by the somewhat brutal architecture of the buildings in Stalin Alley.

The following day we said our goodbyes to Horst, our interpreter who had accompanied us since we arrived in Berlin and whose mastery of a lot of colloquial English had convinced many of us that his claim to have served and fought with the British army following his capture at Alamein was indeed true. We flew out, this time from Temple Hof, catching site of MIG15s on the periphery of the airfield.

Pre-Wedding Preparations

Once back home and after giving a report to my own union branch and also a number of other branches, at the suggestion of the Branch Secretary, I wrote a report for circulation. However the personal reporting combined with the need to earn a living and work on the flat, for which Joan and I had previously collected the key from the landlord, were placing increasing demands upon both of us. After all there are only twenty four hours in a day but even so that did not seem nearly enough for all the things we each needed to do.

By now Jo had really impressed my mother with her knitting skills having the previous Christmas knitted her a cable patterned cardigan. Proudly displaying what her future daughter-on-law could do my mother had received quite a number of orders for sweaters, twin sets, etc., from her friends and also the wives of my father's drinking partners. The money Joan made from making these garments was placed in the pot we had put aside for setting up our home.

In addition to the knitting Joan had also decided to make the bridesmaids' dresses that her blond friend (Joan) and Colleen were to wear at our wedding. One Saturday evening, partly as relaxation from all the work we were both doing which also included delivering the knitwear she had made, we decided to accompany my mother and father on their usual visit to the pub. We entered to find my parents' usual crowd of friends already there and it was actually the first time any of them had actually met Joan who, that evening, was wearing a black pencil skirt, white blouse and stilettos. With her long blue-black hair drawn up in a chignon at the back of her head the whole ensemble emphasised her wonderful figure and stature to perfection.

The women all asked how she managed to stay so slim and the men jokingly told me what a "lucky bugger" I was. After distributing the various knitting commissions she had received Joan was again the subject of much complimentary talk and I could see she was becoming increasingly embarrassed. Then, during a partial lull in the conversations, my attention was drawn to quite a stocky man standing aside from all the others. He was about five feet ten inches tall and appeared to be talking to no-one in particular but loud enough to be heard in general. His remarks were very derogatory and sexist and I suddenly realised they were probably directed at Joan. As I took a step forward my father placed one of his huge hands on my shoulder and pulled me back, stepping past me to approach this man himself. On reaching him, my father grabbed him by the lapels of his jacket with his left hand and hoisted him up into the air, twisting his left wrist as he did so. Then holding him horizontally four feet off the floor, with his right hand threw him straight out onto the pavement with the words "don't you dare talk like that again about my future daughter-in-law".

Joan just stood there open mouthed and shaking then turning to my father asked if the man was going to be alright. My father smiled back at her and told her not to worry on that score; the worst he would suffer would be just a couple of bruises. The landlord of The Swan, Steve Magin, leant across the bar and handed my father a Guinness telling him that he was on the verge of barring that man from the pub as he had been making a real nuisance of himself. He thanked my father and told him they would probably not be seeing him again!

A bit later on, although Jo had become more relaxed I could see she was still shaken by the whole incident so I suggested we call it a night. After saying our goodbyes and with lots of best wishes ringing in our ears and choruses of "we'll see you at the wedding", we took our leave and set off for Vauxhall where, after a prolonged goodnight kiss and caress, we parted.

The following day I was due to install a ring circuit of power points at the flat and Joan had arranged a fitting with Colleen. Bert had kindly volunteered to give us a hand with the decorating, returning a favour I had likewise done for him when I had re-wired a house that Daisy had bought. The ring circuit was a dire necessity in our flat since the only electrics it contained were just two lighting points. This was by no means unusual at that time and indeed quite a few other properties had no electricity supply whatsoever. Older properties in London in the 1950s still tended to have gas lighting. My first experience in electrical work had been the constant re-wiring of fuses at home where my mother would frequently use a multi outlet three which is basically three outlets being used from one lighting point, i.e. one supplying the bulb, the second the radio and the third an iron. If it was cold the outlet for the radio would be replaced by a one bar electric fire which grossly overloaded the fuse box in addition to the added danger from all the trailing leads hanging over the table with no earth protection. However, my continual protests and warnings went unheeded.

It wasn't until the end of my first year of apprenticeship that my parents would allow me to re-wire the house and even then they were initially reluctant to allow me to install twin sockets. They did, however, have the good grace to admit that I had been right when I had carried out the work successfully. It would to drive Joan mad when we later used to visit our respective parents because I always had to take along my tool box as there was inevitably some job or other they would ask me to carry out.

Until I had acquired the knack of hanging wallpaper, under Bert's tutelage, he did the first hanging in our potential home. Like myself he was not overly impressed with the flat's structural integrity and condition. The flat itself consisted of three rooms on the ground floor of a two-storey mid-terrace in a cul-de-sac off the main route down to Clapham Junction, the rail line of which ran to the rear of the terrace. The ceiling in the front room closely resembled a spider's web with its myriad of cracks spreading out to the corners of the room from an ornate central plaster plate. A number of these cracks also ran vertically down the walls to a plaster dado rail and trying to fill them in would be a complete waste of time and effort. No light distemper or the newly introduced emulsion paints would be able to cover them up or hide them. We therefore came up with an idea which our parents thought quite outrageous but our friends thought was truly inspired; we painted it midnight blue and hung an elliptical fluffy yellow fibre glass shade from the pendant in the centre of the ceiling.

With our wedding day fast approaching and our joint saving efforts finally reaching a decent sum, which Joan and I believed would be enough for us to seriously commence window shopping, we began to examine our options. On our frequent visits to the Design Centre in Regent's Street, we had become quite keen with the design simplicity of Scandinavian furniture. We both abhorred what to us was the garish appearance of "G" Plan which was then all the rage. Fortunately, earlier that year, I had worked a stint in the exhibition halls where I had been given some complimentary tickets for the furniture show. It was whilst wandering round the show that we found what we had been looking for; just plain, simple, furniture made from real Afromosia wood with no curves or fancy brass plated embellishments, made by Meredith & Drew, a reputable English manufacturer. We placed an order for a bedroom suite and a dining suite which came at a price our respective parents considered quite outrageous. However, due to Jo's meticulous care and maintenance, fifty years later they are probably worth more now than what we paid then. A kitchen table and four tubular kitchen stools I had made myself, was all we now needed to complete our initial furniture requirements for setting up our first home.

From the £400 we had saved between us we still had enough left to invest in what was to be our one mistake, i.e. a three piece suite purchased from Minty of Oxford. This lasted us a mere five years before it needed to be replaced. Although it proved to be quite comfortable it could not withstand the rigours of the use put upon it by two adults and subsequently two children.

Joan and I were perhaps the first couples to use the idea of drawing up a list with regard to wedding presents, although I have no recollection of using one. My parents bought us a Midwinter Rose dinner set which was always much admired by our guests and is still in good condition today as it was only used on special occasions. Jo's parents bought us a Swedish cutlery set which has similarly survived in good condition which just goes to show that quality counts in the long run. Other than these two items chance had determined we received the linen and utensils we needed.

As our wedding day approached and when I was wandering down Oxford Street one day on my tea break, I happened to bump into a spark I knew. He told me there was the opportunity of a job on the Shell site on the south bank which, he assured me, was a distinct possibility despite the fact that both our names were on a black list being operated by the main electrical contractor on site. He gave me the telephone number of the sub-contractor who had been awarded the contract to install floor trunking. This was a comparatively new form of installation which was, I believe, being used on that site for the first time in the U.K. Having thus sought and been successful in securing a job with this contractor I duly reported on site the following day at 8.00 a.m. I proceeded to a room in the basement of the building which, at that point, had reached a third of its final height. At that time this was the highest paid contracting job in the London area and I was hopeful of the promise of quite a considerable run of well paid employment.

Amongst the thirty or so men present I was amazed to see many faces that I recognised one of whom upon catching my eye scowled and shook his head. Picking up on his warning I merely said "good morning, the name's Tony" and left it at that. After I had satisfied the foreman that I knew what I was doing we all left the basement to proceed to the respective floors that had been allocated to us. I exchanged fraternal greetings with the dozen or so men who, like myself, had all been black listed by Wheelers who were the main electrical contractor.

Two or three days later, on walking back from the portable toilets located at ground level on the site, I was surprised to see emerge from the tower an old adversary of mine, Joe Lee, the Chair of Southwark Trades Council and Central Number One E.T.U. branch. He also happened to be Wheelers' main foreman. Upon recognising me he asked what I was doing on site and two hours later I was told that my services would no longer be required. The other men immediately called a mass meeting of the site's E.T.U. members who approached the Joint Stewards' Committee. The meeting had been set to commence at 1.30 p.m. but needless to say did not take place for the involvement of the joint stewards ensured that an hour after being told I was no longer required it suddenly became imperative that I remain.

Two weeks later, on the Friday afternoon prior to my wedding, a similar situation developed. This time it involved a Plumbing, Heating and Ventilation Engineer and, on this occasion, it was to take longer for the problem to be resolved. All five hundred or so men walked out on strike and work on site immediately ceased.

Our Wedding Day and Start of Married Life

The next morning, following a visit to the barber, I lay soaking in the tin bath in what was referred to as "the laundry". This was located behind the bedroom I shared with my brother Len where my mother, in the mid 1950s, had installed one of the first washing machines available at that time to the working class which she had paid for out of her earnings as a cleaner for the Gas Board. This primitive contraption consisted of a galvanised steel tank with a gas ring in its base. The handle on the tank cover was connected, via a shaft, through the lid to a four bladed paddle in the tank itself. The washing was done by swinging the handle back and forth through an angle of 180° for twenty or thirty minutes. This was a task that usually fell to either myself or Colleen until Lennie was old enough to take this on. On the back of this contraption were a couple of manually operated rollers for wringing out the water from the wet washing once it had gone through the cleaning process. Our mother would then have to negotiate her way through a host of balsa wood model aircraft that were suspended from our bedroom ceiling to collect the laundry and hang it out to dry. The tank of this machine also served to heat the water for the tin bath and I had set this in motion before my visit to the barber so the water would be heated and ready for when I returned.

My toilet complete, I dressed and made my way to the home of John, my Best Man, to make sure he was all suited up and had the rings safely stowed. It being a dull and damp October day I had donned a mock sheepskin jacket to keep my suit dry and presentable. John and I caught a bus and arrived at the church about ten minutes before the wedding was due to start. My brother Len, who was seven years my junior but almost equal in height, was waiting for us at the church door. He assured me that nearly all our expected guests were already inside so handing him my jacket John and I went in.

There was much looking at watches as the start of the ceremony grew near but no sign of Joan. The car, however, was parked outside and Joan's father, Albert, was pleading with her to get out. She had her eyes fixed on Len standing at the church door wearing my jacket and sobbed that "he has changed his mind". From the gestures Albert was making and realising what had happened Len walked over to the car and motioned for Albert to lower the window. Putting his head inside Len said "he's inside you silly bugger".

He then retreated back to the church doorway and signalled the vicar that the bride had arrived. As I turned to see my bride enter the church she absolutely took my breath away. I knew she was beautiful with a great figure but this vision of loveliness advancing down the aisle to take her place at my side was the most beautiful site I have ever seen either before or since.

There was to be another amusing incident barely an hour later when we arrived at the Surrey View Tavern where the reception was being held. Following our arrival Joan and I went upstairs to join our guests. We were later told that as the limousine driver had made his way through the crowded bar he caught sight of my brother, Lennie, and, assuming he was the bridegroom, remarked "he didn't waste much time getting to the bar". Even when he was told that the man standing at the bar was Lennie, the usher, and not the bridegroom the driver still asserted that he was right because he had just driven the bride and groom from the church. My father, however, soon put him right assuring him that Lennie was indeed the usher and the bridegroom's younger brother; he should know because he had made the pair of us! This was a mistake that many other people have made throughout our lives, often mistaking Lennie and myself for each other.

Jo and I had made no plans for a honeymoon and with me now being out on strike we decided to spend our first week together in our flat getting things up together. I was also experiencing some problems with my diabetes during that first week initially due to the high blood sugars resulting from our wedding feast but also the psychological factors from what Spike Milligan used to refer to as "the wedding equipment" not performing because of this. Also, after ten years with diabetes, this symptom could be the first possible indicator of cardio vascular problems. Joan was extremely patient and understanding and at the end of our first week of marriage we succeeded in consummating it. I am pleased to say that this was something we enjoyed together for the next thirty five years, far more frequently than what various surveys reported was the norm for married couples.

At the end of the strike, having achieved our objectives, both Joan and I returned to work. We would travel into Charring Cross by train from Clapham Junction where we would part and proceed separately to our respective destinations. We would likewise meet there at the end of the day for our return journey. Once such evening, packed into a crowded carriage, I became aware of quite a violent and persistent pain in my chest. Joan was becoming ever more concerned and after feeding me with half a tube of extra strong mints with no beneficial effect had to initiate the aid of another passenger to help me off the train. I was certain this was not an insulin reaction and both of them were convinced I was experiencing a heart attack. Luckily, despite the diabetic propensity towards cardio vascular incidents, Jo's suspicions in this regard, and likewise those of the kindly passenger, were subsequently proven not to be correct.

On the concourse of Clapham Station at that time was a chemist where Jo and our kind helper assisted me to enter. At my suggestion the chemist reluctantly prepared a dose of an anti indigestion mixture. His strong inclination was to call a doctor but at my insistence he finally agreed to try my suggestion. A few minutes after swallowing this draught my body at last emitted a hearty burp much to everyone's relief. So, to the cacophony of resounding burps Jo and I walked the half mile home where she immediately went to the kitchen to prepare and cook our evening meal, the vegetables for which I had already prepared prior to our leaving for work that morning.

In addition to all of Joan's other accomplishments, she was also a great cook and, not for the first time, did I tell myself how lucky I was to have such a beautiful and understanding woman in my life. Those early meals far exceeded those of my mother's in respect of taste and variety, yet throughout all of Jo's twenty years of growing up she only had the same ingredients to work with.

That night in bed our love making was frequently interspersed with mention of our earlier pre-dinner scare or giggles at her realisation that one of her legs was still encased in the leg of her pyjamas which, until about a month after our marriage, she had been in the habit of wearing. After this a nightdress became the norm as she soon realised that the warmth generated by cuddling up together was far more satisfying and much less frustrating than having to struggle to release buttons or remove the top or bottom of our respective pyjamas.

The one disturbing factor that was to emerge, although it was not until many years later that we correctly analysed the problem, was that by nature Joan was an owl, taking a long time to relax into sleep. As a consequence she was loathe to wake up in the morning. I, on the other hand, had lark-like tendencies, being able to drop off to sleep relatively easily and ready to go the instant I awoke in the morning. The discipline imposed on my body by the necessity to inject insulin at regular intervals was, I believe, the major factor in all this since on the few occasions I had overslept it was always the case that my sugar levels would be high and not due to nocturnal hypo as the sheets would still be dry.

In those first few weeks of our marriage our different sleep pattern became increasingly clear and it became my habit upon waking to perform a urine test, administer my injection, make the tea and toast and then call Joan for breakfast. Joan would invariably eat her toast but if she was not up by the time it had grown cold I did, in a fit of temper, hurl the piece of toast or indeed the whole loaf across the kitchen or into the bin. Such an unnecessary waste of food has always proved abhorrent to me especially since the onset of my diabetes. So, in order to overcome this, I suggested to Jo that we travel to work separately, meeting up at home in the evening although I would continue to take in her morning cup of tea before I left for work before departing with my customary nudge and goodbye kiss.

Work on the South Bank was now in its final stages and this coincided with some increasing social unrest. The Government had introduced legislation to repeal rent controls in both the public and private sectors. This led to the so-called "St Pancras rent riots". A host of factories, transport depots and building sites, of which the South Bank was one, together with trades unions and tenant bodies, pledged their support to defend tenants from eviction by bailiffs which would be a consequence of this new legislation.

One morning in, I believe the spring of 1961, three women came onto the site and asked to speak to the joint stewards. As a result of this the stewards called a mass meeting which was addressed by two of these women whilst the third and the youngest remained sobbing in the background. With anger mounting significantly amongst the men who were listening, they were told about a party of bailiffs who, escorted by a large body of police, had that morning broken through a cordon of pickets that had been set up by the tenants of Council flats in St Pancras. With the use of considerable force they had evicted the young woman, who was pregnant with her third child, together with her two other children. They had then proceeded to empty the flat of all their possessions, some of which were simply thrown over the third floor balcony to crash to the ground below. As a result this family was now homeless.

With a roar of rage those at the meeting determined they would march to the scene of this diabolical outrage and make their cause and intention known to as many of their compatriots on other sites as possible. This resulted some two hours later in thousands of workers in the building trades marching at least ten abreast down Oxford Street. It was here that I witnessed one of the best examples of quick thinking that I have ever seen. As has always been the case, whenever workers unite to demonstrate any authoritarian opposing force, usually with a police acquiescence attempt to disrupt them, on this occasion every one hundred yards along Oxford Street a thickset and sometimes tall figure stood yelling racist taunts and slogans. After a while this became too much for one of our E.T.U. colleagues amongst us who caught hold of the bell of the megaphone one of these louts was using but instead of wresting it off him, as we all anticipated, he pulled it forward and rammed it back hard into his teeth. The ranks behind us passed that spot undisturbed thereafter.

A couple of months after this incident saw the completion of the Shell tower as it reached its final height. A friend of mine, a West Indian man named Dave, having recently arrived in the U.K., asked me if I would point out to him the sights. So we ascended to the roof of the lift motor room where we stood at 417 feet on what was then the tallest building in London. Dave was clutching my shoulders in some trepidation and standing in a slight breeze I pointed out as many sites and buildings of interest that I could make out between the Thames Estuary and Heathrow, both of which were just perceptible.

One evening I invited Dave to spend the evening with us and he showed Joan and I some photographs of his wife and three children that had been taken in their home which I believe was Trinidad. He was a skilled cabinet maker and the furniture we could see in those photographs was absolutely beautiful. We were shocked to realise that it could only be innate prejudice against his colour that forced this extraordinary skilled craftsman to accept the semi-skilled role of electrician's mate. Jo urged me to do whatever I could to find the address of the National Union of Furniture Trades to locate the name of a possible contact therein. Dave was delighted and even bought a bunch of flowers which he asked me to give to Joan on his behalf. Sadly I lost contact with him not long after this as the contract I was working on over on the South Bank came to an end.

One unexpected outcome of Dave's visit occurred a couple of days later. A small cul-de-sac named Shelgate Road located off the main drag, contained about twenty terraced houses on each side. Those on the opposite side to us were occupied exclusively by white families. On our side of the block there were two black families, one living next door to us and the other at the main road end of the terrace. It always struck us as odd that during the time we were refurbishing our flat, whenever we had said good morning or good afternoon, the only response we received was a perplexed look or an embarrassed smile and nod of the head. However if any white people happened to be outside there would be glares and frequent grunts of discontent from them at our attempts at friendly greetings.

Much to our surprise, the day after Dave's visit, it being a nice Saturday morning when we were making our way to the shops, we actually exchanged names with our black neighbours and were even introduced to their children. They explained their initial reluctance to respond to our former greetings. Having noticed Dave arrive at our flat the previous evening they had kept an eye out for him leaving being concerned for his safety. He had apparently reassured them on this score. For the six months or so that Joan and I lived in that flat we never, after that, ever received anything other than glares from the white residents with the exception of the seventeen year old lad and his mother who occupied the flat above ours.

The state of interracial relations in London at the beginning of the 1960s was not good, to say the least, yet on the sites on which I worked I never witnessed anything other than harmony. However, having said, that I am white so therefore, I suppose, not really in a position to judge.

It was common practise even then, when filling out application forms, to find questions regarding nationality but not ethnicity since that, for the most part, was obvious. On one occasion when I was completing one such form and thinking what the hell difference did it make provided I could do the job, I wrote Chinese Eskimo. The recipient of my form merely rolled his eyes and told me to start the following morning!

That particular job was on St James' Hospital which was about two miles away from where I lived and only ten minutes or so by bike. It was also a useful location in the event I had any problems in relation to my diabetes. A problem did occur just a few days later although not in relation to my condition. This was one of the very few sites where it was possible to use an electric drill and while I was drilling into a rusty girder a flake of rust became embedded in my eye causing considerable discomfort. After having it removed I had to wear a patch over that eye for a few days.

On the morning I had the patch removed I saw one of the most amazing sights I have ever seen. We had entered a service duct under the main ward block to check some armoured cables and were using a Tilly Lamp for illumination. After we had checked about thirty yards of this duct I noticed the wall appeared to be rippling. My first thought was that my eye was perhaps still affected by the treatment and my second thought was that this illusion was some strange new reaction to the insulin. However my mate with whom I was working assured me that he had also noticed this anomaly so we walked on to check if the same thing happened further along. Finding this to be the case we held the Tilly Lamp close to the wall and discovered, to our amazement and horror, that the movement was being caused by a seething mass of albino cockroaches. They must have been that colour either because they lived in total darkness or they had some strange chameleon-like ability to change colour to match the white washed walls. The gas lighter I had used ten years earlier to burn the cockroaches off the walls in St Giles, would have been useless here where nothing short of a full scale military flame thrower would have made any impression. I believe the hospital has since been rebuilt and I sincerely hope the new one does not have a similar problem!

About a week or so later I was due to spend a week at Southsea attending the annual E.T.U. Policy Conference so I decided to book a double room so that Jo could join me on the Friday night for the Civic Reception which would be a pleasant night out for us. She had arranged to see the doctor on the preceding Wednesday and, if our suspicions proved correct, we would have cause to celebrate.

In the event, that week proved to be quite momentous. Firstly we received the news that we had been awarded a 4d (roughly 2p today) an hour wage increase taking us to the premier position in the building trade in relation to wages. Secondly, in moving the branch's resolution that I had drawn up following the visit to the D.D.R. the previous year, I had addressed and received unanimous support from the seven hundred delegates in attendance. I had also received compliments from Frank Haxell, Frank Foulks and Ted Hill, the Boilermaker Leader. I had succeeded in keeping both my nerves and my diabetes under control.

Therein lies the secret of carbohydrate control and once one understands the basic 5gm portion of the different carbohydrates it is easy to develop an innate ability to look at foods such as pastry, rice, or potatoes and judge how much you need. It is a complete fallacy to think that every time you need to eat all your food has to be weighed. It is certainly true that you need to do so now and then to double check that your judgement is correct but experience and common sense in this regard is very quickly acquired. The medical profession will constantly warn you of complications that can result from your condition but by strict observance of the need to balance diet, insulin and exercise, these problems can be avoided and are by no means inevitable. I would advise anyone with this condition to do as I was advised and learn from your own experiences and those of other Type One diabetics and become your own expert. You too can lead a fulfilled life.

Joan duly arrived on the Friday afternoon dressed in a light blue linen box jacket suit she had recently bought. She looked stunning. I met her at the station and we walked to the lodgings I had pre-booked. She teased me with regard to her news for which she knew I was anxiously awaiting, not saying a word till we reached our destination. Once there the landlady offered to make us a cup of tea which she would bring up to us, expressing her hope that we would find the bed comfortable. This was said with a knowing smile to which Joan responded she was sure we would but could the landlady delay the tea until a bit later.

Once in our room Joan gave me the news that I was to be a father, she was three months pregnant. I was overjoyed. She also told me that she had asked the doctor if it was safe to continue our marital relations whose response was that it would be OK until she found it too uncomfortable and that no harm would befall the baby. With an impish grin she removed her jacket and said "shall we see if he is right?" I did not need a second invitation and could not shed my clothes quick enough for we had not seen each other for four whole days.

Later, when we joined the landlady downstairs and had enjoyed a nice cup of tea, she turned to the pair of us and with a knowing smile looked at Joan and said "you're pregnant aren't you?" Joan responded that she was and asked her how she knew. The landlady replied that she could see it in her eyes and face and asked if I was as happy about it as she was. Puzzled I beamed at her, realising that it was perhaps not quite so obvious from my face. It was only with increased maturity that I came to recognise the look that the landlady back then had so quickly recognised herself.

At around 6.30 p.m. that evening and having completed our preparatory washing, dressing, etc., with the room and street keys safely in our possession we left for the Southsea Guildhall Reception, eagerly anticipating the dance that would follow. With the reception and speeches over we entered the large hall where the delegates and their wives were either seated at the bar or already on the dance floor dancing to the live band that was on the stage. Joan indicated that, rather than her usual Babycham, she would like a pint of shandy so I made my way over to the bar. I had also decided that rather than the pipe I usually smoked I would have a cigar and somewhat to my surprise Joan said she would have one too instead of her usual cigarette. When I asked her if she was sure her response was "if it's good enough for you, it's good enough for me". When some of the other wives present queried her with regard to her choice of cigar and pint of shandy her response was the same as the one she gave to me, "if it's OK for him, it's OK for me".

Always capable of standing up for herself and others, Joan was a firm believer in equality between the sexes and equal rights in all spheres. She was way ahead of the feminism to emerge twenty years later and indeed in the 1980s, would frequently cite that she regarded the pursuit of feminism far less important than the pursuit of what she termed "real" equality. I suppose to some degree her approach was clearly demonstrated that evening in 1961 in Southsea.

We arrived home the following day to find a letter waiting for us the contents of which were a big contributor in making that past week one of the best we ever had in our many years together. It came from the Department of Employment advising that under the Industrial Housing Scheme there was a possible vacancy for an electrician in Swindon, Wiltshire. If I submitted an application which was accepted then we would be provided with Local Authority housing.

This was great news for us, particularly in light of the fact that a week or so earlier we had experienced a very worrying and potentially dangerous incident when Joan had been sitting at our dining table using her sewing machine. This was an early Singer hand operated one as opposed to the more usual treadle variety. Years earlier this had been passed on to Joan from her grandmother, a miner's wife and a really grand old lady. It was from her that Joan had learned her initial knitting, dressmaking and cooking skills which she had so ably perfected.

From memory I believe Joan was adjusting the length of some curtains that either her grandmother or mother had sent to us. Jo had drawn my attention to the dust that was falling on the material and being a bit dubious I stood back across the room and although the light was on I got a torch and a tea cloth. Puzzled Jo asked me what I was doing and watched as I hung the tea towel over the lampshade to stop the upward glow from the light and then shone the torch onto the ceiling above where she was sitting. I then asked her to start sewing and as she spun the handle of the machine I could see flakes of blue drifting down from the ceiling. Suddenly concerned I instructed her to stop and stepping forward I lifted the sewing machine and the material off the table and asked her to spread a couple of blankets over the table whilst I fetched a broom. Having done as I had asked she wanted to know what the broom was for, following which I proceeded to show her. I held the handle above my head and gingerly tapped the end against the ceiling above, where just minutes before, she had been sitting. The effect was just the same as putting your finger into a spider's web. A piece of the ceiling about the size of a dustbin lid fell in thousands of small fragments onto the blanket that was protecting the table. This was followed by a cloud of very ancient plaster dust. The only thing that had been holding all this in place had been the three coats of midnight blue paint we had applied in our efforts to hide the network of cracks streaking across the ceiling.

I silently gave thanks that Joan had drawn my attention to the dust and she now worriedly asked me what were going to do about this. I said we were going to do nothing. The landlord was going to have the whole ceiling re-plastered before the weekend or I would get the Building Inspector to deal with it. Upon that I went out to a telephone box and rang the landlord, relating to him the details of what had just occurred. I did, however, leave out the bit about tapping the ceiling with the broom handle. I told him this incident was extremely unlikely to have been the result of any vibrations emanating from the sewing machine but was wholly down to his failure to check and replaced the ceiling years before. Luckily he conceded defeat and two days later, using the same method I had, the plasterers bought down and replaced the whole ceiling.

Joan was both relieved, and I think impressed, with the way I had handled the whole thing. We now had a brand new white ceiling albeit still with eighteen inches of midnight blue on the walls between the paper and the ceiling. As things turned out, however, this was of no consequence for within a matter of months my application under the Industrial Housing Scheme proved successful and we moved to Swindon.

Around the time of our wedding Colleen had started courting a young man named Ron who, like myself, was a keen cyclist. Unfortunately Colleen was no more adept at cycling than Joan. Ron had bought a Vespa Scooter and not being able to afford to buy a new one I asked him if he could keep his eye open for a second hand model for myself. The four of us become close friends and we all looked forward to being able to venture out of London together at weekends.

I duly acquired an N.S.U. Prima which in appearance resembled a Lambreta rather than a Vespa, i.e. it had no bulbous blisters encasing the engine. Aside from a slight argument with a "Keep Left" bollard I soon mastered riding the scooter sufficient to suggest a trip down to Swindon where I was due to attend an interview one Saturday morning. My slight mishap had resulted in a bent leg shield and a severe warning from the police. If my interview proved successful it would then leave us the afternoon in which to explore what would potentially become our new home town.

Joan was sceptical that we would be able to manage such a journey in just one day and it was not until I had persistently protested that we could easily manage it that it suddenly dawned on her I was referring to Swindon, in Wiltshire and not Swinton in Lancashire as she had originally thought. So with panniers packed with sandwiches and flasks of tea and coffee, on what turned out to be a bright and sunny day, the four of us set off keeping in mind that my interview was scheduled for 12.00 noon.

The journey went well apart from one minor scare for Joan and myself. Having left the A4 we got onto the road that passed through Chiltern Foliat which had a sharp right turn onto a single lane bridge over the river Kennet. Ron was out in front and travelling quite fast and as he lined up his Vespa to take the bend he held up his right hand in warning. I dropped my speed and after taking a quick look round the bend immediately chickened out of attempting it and went straight on down what I believe was a private road where I stopped, turned round and took what was now the left turn over the bridge. On catching sight of the bridge and its stone walls Joan had increased her already tight grip on my waist. Having caught up with Ron and Colleen she relaxed her grip and we proceeded at a more leisurely pace.

As we crested Liddington Hill we saw spread out in front of us a town that was somewhat larger than I had anticipated given the impression of it I had received four years earlier when I had first glimpsed it at midnight through a train window. As we crossed the Coate Water roundabout unto Queens Drive I was amazed to see extensive building work underway on both the left (private) and right (Council) hand sides. It crossed my mind that this was probably the reason the town needed electricians and the thought of a future confined to wiring houses filled me with dread. On reaching the end of Queens Drive we stopped and parked up on a wide expanse of grass in order to eat our lunch. I passed on my apprehensions to the others and Joan, bless her, told me to turn down any job offer if my fears proved to be correct.

The interview took place in Old Town above a shop retailing in radios and televisions. However my earlier apprehensions were soon set aside as I was informed that they were looking to appoint electricians with extensive experience, particularly in industrial installation work. Suitably reassured, despite my age which was just approaching my twenty third birthday, I confirmed that I was suitably qualified and held a City & Guilds Certificate in installation work. The demeanour of the man interviewing me markedly changed after that and it was now myself who was in the driving seat. The first thing I wanted to establish was the exact nature of the work on offer, the second being the hourly rate of pay and finally the accommodation arrangements prior to the Local Authority's offer being available. He grimaced when I announced that I was not prepared to settle for anything less than the pay rates I was getting in London together with the full cost of the lodgings being covered. The offer on the table was a room in a local hotel on a bed and breakfast basis with a daily meal allowance and a rate of pay equal to that I was getting in London, plus removal costs when Local Authority accommodation became available. In the absence of children this would be a two bedroom flat in approximately three to four weeks' time. The work involved would be the installation of an electrical supply to the "C" building on the Pressed Steel

Fisher car body plant site. So with all the arrangements made and the relevant expenses secured I agreed to start on the following Thursday. Before I left the building I tipped off another couple of men who were waiting outside for their interviews with regard to making sure they likewise mentioned the London rate.

On re-joining Joan, Colleen and Ron, we all then left to explore the town and were taken aback at the extent of house building taking place and the seeming lack of any obvious factories in the immediate area. Following our tour we then departed for home and I proposed using the expenses I had received on a dinner of spaghetti bolognese that evening at one of the numerous coffee bars that were then sprouting like mushrooms across the inner London area.

Start of our New Life and Family in Swindon

In the three weeks before I received my letter confirming our accommodation, each morning before going across to the hotel for breakfast the men would gather in the shop doorway trying to ascertain whether any of the mail lying on the floor contained our respective names, arriving as it did between 7.00 and 7.15 a.m. None of us liked the separation from our wives and families and were for ever speculating how far from the top of the housing list we were and whether the accommodation offered to us would be old or new build.

Work wise, a couple of amusing incidents occurred. Just outside the entrance to the site on Swindon Road was an old cottage with a large garden surrounded by a metre high stone wall on which we would sit and eat our lunch. On one such occasion when I was sitting there I became aware that my half eaten sandwich was being tugged and on looking over, to my surprise, I saw a large pig trying to pull it out of my hand. As the pig was a darn site bigger than me I very quickly released my grip rather than try to wrestle my sandwich from the jaws of one very determined pig which would clearly have been counter productive, diabetes wise. So reluctantly accepting the loss of my lunch I wandered down the road to a local store where I bought an eccles cake and a pint of milk. When I related this incident to Joan at the weekend she found it highly amusing.

The second amusing incident occurred later at work when we were installing a very large trunking system in the roof of "C" building. A colleague was attempting to balance an elongated elbow of this trunking on the table of a radial drill to open up the holes in the flange of the elbow. With the obvious danger of the drill snatching or jamming this was clearly a two-man job. I therefore went to his assistance and proceeded to hold and manoeuvre the elbow between the holes. As this operation was in progress a man unknown to either of us in a very authoritarian voice told me to return to my own job. I pointed out to him that I would be doing so once the flange was finished. Then with heavy emphasis he said that he had told me to go. When I asked him who he was he replied that his name was Penfold and he was the foreman at Pressed Steel. I responded that as I was employed by the electrical contractors he had no jurisdiction over me and repeated what I had said earlier that I would return to my own job when the flange was safely done. If he wished to interfere with our schedules then I advised him to contact our foreman. An hour or so later our foreman, who had been in Swindon for about three years after coming down from Birmingham, told me that I had to leave the site.

Another of our men who was nearby overheard this command and within fifteen minutes our foreman was informed that if I was sent off site then the rest of my colleagues would be going with me. He was quite shaken by this announcement, having had no experience of the solidarity commonly displayed among the London sparks. He decided he should contact our office and in the meantime asked us all to return to work to await any further developments which we agreed to do. In the meantime we were contacted by the P.S.F. sparks who told us that as a result of a recent full plant dispute there were a number of T.G.W.U., A.E.U. and E.T.U. men who had been blacklisted and their fate was currently being discussed at national level but they remained outside so advised us to look for a compromise solution.

The next morning it was suggested by management that I undertake the installation of the outside lighting for the building next door which was the Deloro Stellite site. After carrying out an initial examination I estimated there to be about a month's work so I agreed. My fellow work mates accepted my decision with some reluctance, pointing out that it did not resolve the issue of jurisdiction. Our employer, fearful of its future standing with Pressed Steel Fisher, nevertheless undertook to advise them that their employees were their concern alone. With this compromise achieved I spent three pleasant weeks in the sunshine connecting up street lamps whilst the other men sweated under a glass roof installing trunking without interference from the management at Pressed Steel.

A couple of weeks later I received a key to a two bedroom flat in a three storey block on the Penhill estate. So, armed with several sheets of graph paper and a twenty five feet rule, I made an inspection of the property and a drawing which I could show to Joan at the weekend. I was careful not to forget to include window measurements, as she had previously instructed. Joan was delighted with the flat but also a little disappointed that we would have to wait for the birth of a second child before we would qualify for a house. However she pulled herself up and remarked that we had not even had our first one yet and asked me if I wanted a boy or a girl. I responded that it made no difference to me as long as they were both O.K. and that nature would determine the sex. I added that we would both accept nature's decision to which she responded that we had no alternative now whilst she stroked her ever growing stomach.

A fortnight later we moved into our flat, thrilled to have hot running water and, for me at least, my first experience of the pleasure of lying in a six feet enamel bath as opposed to a tin one just four feet in length which was a bit of a squeeze for one such as I with a six feet, one and a half inch frame.

Joan and I measured up our furniture and cut out cardboard shapes from an old cereal packet to represent the various pieces. From drawings I had made on graph paper we determined which pieces of furniture would best suit each room. Pleased with our efforts in that regard Joan then turned her attention to the curtains.

We duly made arrangements for our move to Swindon, much to the sadness of our respective parents who were finding it difficult to accept the fact, particularly our mothers. In addition to both of us having left our family homes we were now going to move to Swindon, some ninety miles distant. In hindsight, rather rashly, we did point out that our flat had two bedrooms which meant either set of parents could come and stay with us on a visit sometimes.

Two weeks later Joan and I were settled into our flat and had registered with the local G.P. Having also met our neighbours we started to adjust to the town and our new surroundings. Around this time something very odd occurred. Together with one of my colleagues, both of us party members, I made contact with the local C.P. Branch Secretary by the name of Ike and he asked if either of us could do some wiring in his house. As I had now finished my job on the street lights and therefore in need of further work I agreed that I could do it.

Ike gave me the money for the materials I would need and I set off for the local wholesaler. After I had given my order at the counter the telephone in the office at the back started to ring. The young man who had taken my order momentarily left the counter to answer it and on returning asked me if my name was Huzzey. When I asked him why, to my astonishment, he said the call was for me. I responded that it couldn't be for me as I had only lived in Swindon for a month and nobody knew me so rather bemusedly I asked him the name of the caller. He said it was someone called Cecil Ferris. Even more bemused I said "who the hell is he; I don't know any Cecil?" The young man replied "well he has asked for you by name so you had better ask him". On taking the call I was asked if I would be able to go to an address the location of which was only about five minutes away so, having nothing, to lose I agreed.

When I arrived at the address I had been given I was surprised to find it was an electrical contractors where I was told to go upstairs as I was expected. In something of a daze and not knowing what to expect, I proceeded up a narrow wooden staircase to the landing above off of which were two doors, one on either side. Not quite knowing which one to choose I followed my natural inclination and knocked on the door to the left and was beckoned to "come in". I entered to find a short wirey framed man, whom I estimated to be in his early fifties, sitting behind a desk. He introduced himself as the Cecil Ferris of the phone call I had received and waved for me to sit down. He then excused himself while he asked for his brother, Gerald, to come in. Moments later another man around the same age and height but of Pickwickian proportions came into the room and sat down in a third chair.

Cecil then turned to me and said that he understood I had recently been laid off by Hickmans and he wanted me to know they were considering backing me if I decided that I would like to take the matter further which struck me as a very strange proposition. Only being used to the machinations and practises of large firms I had no knowledge of the practices of small town Chambers of Commerce. I was somewhat amazed at the apparent willingness of these two brothers to commit their firm to financing on my behalf any legal action I considered taking with regard to my recent lay off and this apparent suggestion had me quite baffled.

I asked them how they had been able to locate me at the wholesalers I had just been visiting where Cecil had contacted me by telephone. I was told that I had been seen entering the building and they had taken the opportunity to contact me there. I thought for a moment that I was becoming paranoid and wanted to know who on earth would know me let alone report my presence and to what purpose. I felt this was ridiculous even knowing that I had been drawn to the attention of Special Branch some two years previously. My only response was that I would think about it.

In the meantime however these brothers were prepared to offer me a job which, at that stage, would be house wiring on a new estate. With a new baby on the way I knew I needed the work so I accepted their offer on the understanding that should something come up that was more suited to my experience with either themselves or another firm then I would be taking that. They both agreed to this and emphasised it was my industrial and commercial experience plus my qualifications they were interested in. It dawned on me that these two men seemed to know far more about me than I was comfortable with and I wondered if Ike, who was a respected local Headmaster, had approached them perhaps calling in a past favour. However when I later asked him if this was the case he vigorously denied it pointing out, quite reasonably, that he knew nothing of my previous experience or academic background.

To this day I still wonder how all this came about and the only clue I ever received was from one of the other sparks in the firm who told me the brothers had been quite taken aback when Hickmans had won the contract for the electrical installation in the Pressed Steel Fisher "C" building. Rather surprisingly they had succeeded in beating the Ferris Brothers for this contract, who were an old established firm.

In their view, Hickmans was an upstart mob which came into existence when a local hotelier had bought out the radio and television supplier and opened an electrical contracting operation. Their success had been the result of a time and material clause which was a means of solely screwing up costs for work, outside or extra to that in the original spec. This practice was common with metropolitan contractors as I well knew but at that time apparently new to Swindon.

However whilst this may very well have explained the brothers' preparedness to potentially finance a legal action on my behalf it did not explain the origin of the phone call I had received whilst I was at the wholesalers. With regard to legal action I knew there were no grounds to pursue such a case since having finished the street lighting there had been nothing further for me to do electrically on that site, therefore negating the need for me to remain. I never did discover who had seen me enter the wholesalers and subsequently report the sighting to the two brothers.

Following those Saturday morning interviews in June, the three of us who had started working in Swindon at the same time had each applied to transfer from our respective E.T.U. branches to the one in Swindon. Over the course of the last three or four years the size of this branch had doubled its membership due mainly to the increased requirement for electricians in the rail workshops. This coincided with the switch from steam to diesel powered locomotives with three coach multiple units. Most of these workers came from contracting in London.

This increase in membership considerably changed the character and outlook of the branch from a somewhat parochial laid back body to one that was more pro-active and broader based. This resulted in an internecine struggle for position. In order to initiate a transfer between branches the Branch Secretary had to ensure that members were in compliance, i.e. up-to-date with membership contributions, and not subject to any charges under Union rules. My own Branch Secretary provided me with a glowing letter of recommendation setting out my record within the Union and citing the branch's regret at losing me which, in their opinion, was Swindon's gain. In extreme embarrassment I had to sit in front of my new branch members and listen whilst this glowing accolade was read out. Unfortunately this brought about unforeseen and unfortunate consequences. The struggle for power within the branch was in relation to the post of Branch Secretary and the main contender was a man called Danny Lee. Thinking I was a potential rival he was not too pleased to accept me into the branch which led to a somewhat guarded working relationship between us in all future Union affairs. Whilst we invariably agreed on policy, agreement on tactics and strategy in achieving given objectives was always a contentious issue. Danny was then a steward and later convenor of the electricians employed within the rail works and I had to give him his due when I was also recruited into the factory and became Chair of the Joint Shops' Committee.

My job of house wiring continued into the New Year giving me more than a passing acquaintance with the glutinous waterlogged nature of the Swindon soil which, on numerous occasions saw me with about fifty six pounds of clay stuck to each boot when attempting to get into a half constructed house, i.e. no floor. This continual struggle to move between one pair of semi-detached houses to another invariably brought on a hypo and I had to stuff myself with glucose.

Joan, meanwhile, as the baby grew in her womb, was getting increasingly fed up of having to wear trousers with even larger waistbands. Before her pregnancy I had been able to encircle her waist in my two hands and the ends of my thumbs and forefingers were able to meet comfortably without squeezing. Appalled at the cost of maternity wear and with winter approaching she had bought some suitably warm and durable material and a paper pattern and, despite the scepticism of our respective mothers, made herself a maternity suite with an expanding adjustable front panel. However, the skill involved in making this together with the end result impressed them both and again brought home to me just how lucky I had been to fall in love with such a lovely and accomplished girl.

As the time for the birth of the baby grew closer it became clear that it would be at least another twelve to fifteen months before my name would come to the top of the list for work at the Union controlled rail works which was by far the highest earner for electricians at that time. In the meantime I started to look for a means of escape from the monotony of house wiring. This led me to approach a non-Union firm named Linton & Hirst who had recently relocated from London following a dispute. A few discrete white lies secured me a place as their second maintenance spark, the first having transferred with them. I began this job in January 1962 and sought and gained their agreement to my taking two days off when Joan went into labour.

At the insistence of our parents we had had a telephone installed, as had they. In the 1960s it was quite rare for the "working class" to have telephones and in January 1961, with a population of some eight million or so, there were only two Huzzeys in the London directory, these being my father and my uncle Charles.

At about 10.00 p.m. on the 21st February, prompted by some slight niggling discomfort, Joan and I went to bed. By 12.00 o'clock these niggles had increased to much sharper pains every ten minutes or so. Some months earlier, much to the concern of our mothers, we had been told that Joan would have a home confinement. She had been seeing a midwife for the past couple of months in order to prepare herself for what to expect. When she had told the midwife that I intended to be present at the birth, which was what she wanted, the midwife had, with some reluctance, agreed.

In 1961 home births in Swindon were frequent but the presence of the fathers at the birth was not generally encouraged. However Joan and I were determined that I should be there. The midwife had instructed me to call her when the pains were coming at twenty minute intervals so I had called her when they had started. After the midwife came, and some two hours later following a further examination of Joan, she told us that she felt this was going to be a long delivery. However she sought to reassure us that everything was progressing normally and it was Joan's "un-pregnant" slimness that would cause the delay.

With increasing anxiety I sat with Joan who continuously squeezed my hand with desperate pressure as the frequency and intensity of the pains increased. The midwife finally issued instructions for her to push, now also attended by the G.P. who had had to make a cut to ease the birth canal. Finally, after eighteen hours of unremitting pain and effort, the crown of our baby's head appeared. By this time I was feeling very guilty at being the cause of such suffering to my beautiful wife.

At last, with one mighty push, our baby was born. At the site of so much blood and what I can only describe as a mixture of yellow and brownish goo, I looked in alarm at the midwife. As she lifted the baby clear the doctor tied off and cut the cord and both looked at my worried face. The midwife then proceeded to wash the baby and turning to me announced that we had a perfectly normal baby girl and congratulated us on the birth of our daughter. I let out a whoop of relief and delight as she handed the baby to Joan who managed a smile of relief at the end of her pain and also of complete joy as she held our first born child who we named Dawn. As I bent over and gently kissed her I knew then that nothing life could ever throw at us, short of death, would ever take me away from my family and to hell with the diabetes; there was no way I was going to fail them.

Joan soon dropped off into an exhausted and well earned sleep and Dawn was passed to her proud father to hold whilst the midwife prepared her crib. Like her mother, Dawn was now fast asleep. The doctor then advised me that he would return the following morning to stitch the small cut he had made and instructed me not to forget to eat. I temporarily retired to the kitchen to make a sandwich where I was joined by the midwife. Although Joan had chosen to breastfeed, the midwife ran through the preparation of bottles and, using a dummy baby doll, instructed me how to put on a nappy. Following a few attempts I finally managed this to her satisfaction. She then left assuring me that she would be a regular visitor but to call her if I needed to.

The first telephone calls however were to both sets of Dawn's grandparents who were obviously delighted to receive the news of her birth. When told that his granddaughter had been born at 2.00 p.m. my father, with a choked voice, said "Dawn arrives late in your house, that's what you get for moving west"! Joan's mother, Isobel arrived the next day to find me up to my elbows at the kitchen sink washing nappies. Whilst she was impressed at my efforts I got a telling off for using the kitchen sink instead of the bath. Although I had apparently done very well she announced that she would take over and I could return to work.

Of the three of us who had started working in Swindon the wife of one of the other men was also pregnant with their third child. This was again to be a home delivery but was sadly not to be a successful one as the baby was breach and tragically died. Whilst the wife was fortunately physically OK the same could obviously not be said psychologically.

The wife of the third of us, under the so-called wives tale of "new house, new baby" sure enough became pregnant with their second child within a month of moving to Swindon. The three wives soon became friends and one evening I called round to see one of my friends, called Arthur, to discuss a problem I was having with our scooter. This I had parked to the left of their front door so that we could examine the engine. His wife Karlen[5] was leaning out of an upstairs window to ask how we were getting on just as I was attempting to start it. The scooter had an electric starter which was started by turning the key. Initially it did not fire but with a sudden bang the spark plug flew out of the cylinder head straight up into the air narrowly missing Karlen's head. Though shocked she assured us she was fine but the incident had certainly

5   Karlen was the daughter of Harry Francis, General Secretary of the British Musicians Union and it was reputed that her name was made up from the first three letters of the Christian names of Karl Marx and Vladimir Lenin

scared the living daylights out of me. I fully expected her to miscarry but thankfully she gave birth to a healthy baby three months later. Arthur and I did, however, manage to solve the problem with my scooter which turned out to be the thread in the cylinder head which had given out.

I had been toying with the idea of getting a motorbike capable of having a sidecar fitted to it and now decided it was time to start looking for one. So I contacted one of my electrician colleagues in the rail works, Alan, who was not only an outstanding mechanic but was also himself a keen trail rider and cross country sidecar racer. He very soon found a suitable machine for me, an MSS Velocette, which was the workhorse version of a renowned racing bike, the Viper. Alan undertook to ensure the bike was in good working order and proceeded to strip and rebuild it for me.

By now Dawn was making good progress and was now nearing six months old. Wanting to show her off to her former work colleagues, Joan planned to journey to London for a couple of days where she would also visit her respective aunts and uncles. One evening whilst she was away I decided that I would accompany three of the men with whom I worked at Linton & Hirst on a bike ride. We had all progressed onto owning and riding more powerful machines.

One of these, our sparks' mate named Brian, was the father of three young children and had recently progressed from riding a moped to a motorbike which had a sidecar attached. Trevor was single and the same age as myself and was the only really experienced rider among us, riding a BSA Gold Star. He was an orphan having lost his parents in the Canvey Island floods in 1952. The third of our number was Bill, a local man and another expectant father who had expressed a desire to accompany us. Trevor and I suggested he sit in the sidecar as this would assist in ensuring the third wheel of the unit would remain stable on the ground. He reluctantly agreed and we all set off after work one evening with the intention of riding down to Cirencester and returning via Chippenham.

Although we were travelling a little too fast for my liking, averaging around 70 mph, things went well until we reached Cirencester. It does take a little while to become adept at handling a bike with a sidecar attached but in spite of this Brian was still travelling in front of me riding at my own pace at the rear of our little convoy. On reaching our intended goal, the others had all stopped in Cirencester allowing me time to catch them up and also check our intended route back which, at my suggestion, was the one Joan and I had travelled when we had ridden down on the scooter through the Stroud Valley. It was here that I raised my concerns over our speed which Brian did not appear to take too seriously insisting that he had mastered the machine and that everything was OK. However both Trevor and I thought he was being too over confident, bearing in mind he was also carrying Bill in the sidecar which was holding it down. Announcing that he was finding riding in the sidecar to be too claustrophobic the two men decided they would continue with the next stage of our journey with Bill riding pillion. Thus we carried on with Trevor again leading and our speed now tempered to around 60 mph.

A few miles outside of Cirencester the road contained a left hand bend followed almost immediately by a bend to the right running down hill. As I manoeuvred the first of these bends I caught sight of a shoe lying in the centre of the road and instinctively dropped my speed. Then, halfway round the second bend, I saw the remains of the sidecar buried under the front nearside wheels of a loaded flat-bed truck. Absolutely horrified I pulled over and looked around desperately for signs of Bill and Brian. Not being able to see either of them I crossed the road and caught sight of Trevor about thirty yards away standing shivering and sobbing at the rear of the truck. On the verge behind him lay Brian spread eagled for all the world like a pinned out frog, almost certainly dead. Of Bill, however, there was no immediate sign but I eventually caught sight of him lying on the edge of a ditch at the bottom of which ran a steady stream of water. He was very clearly badly injured but thankfully still breathing. He was also in imminent danger of rolling into the ditch but fortunately the truck driver had the presence of mind to position himself alongside him to ensure he did not slide down as Trevor was in no fit state to do so.

I rushed off to locate a telephone box or a house with a telephone to call the emergency services. Some time later an ambulance arrived on the scene and took both men to Cirencester Hospital where Brian was pronounced dead on arrival and Bill died in the early hours of the following morning.

Trevor and I went back to my empty flat where, at my insistence, after a few drinks to steady our nerves, he spent the night sleeping on the living room floor. He told me that he had caught sight of the combination and truck in his wing mirror and as Brian and Bill had come round the bend the wheel of the sidecar had lifted resulting in the whole unit being thrown off balance leaving Brian with no option but to steer straight across the path of the oncoming truck. Although the driver of the truck had braked heavily he could not avoid the resultant collision.

The following morning when we went to work our concerns were solely with the families of our lost colleagues. One of the tool makers, who was an A.E.U. member, together with myself and one of our female colleagues came up with a scheme which we hoped would raise some money for the two families. About sixty percent of the total staff were female, working in either the catering section, clerical staff or machine operatives. The money raising scheme we devised, after discussing it with our respective work mates, was based on pontoon and the football league and we hoped that once established it would be ongoing. Everyone wishing to take part would pay 30p each week and the money raised would be split with 10% going to the winner, 60% to Brian's widow and three children, and the remaining 30% to Bill's widow. With the exception of one member of the management team, everyone signed up, totalling around two hundred people. When my job at the plant came to an end and I left this workplace some three months later the scheme was still up and running.

I was determined that Joan and Dawn would not be placed in a similar tragic situation so I purchased a second hand sidecar and chassis in which I placed a one hundred weight bag of cement, practising driving the whole rig till I felt confident in my ability to handle it safely.

By now my name had reached the top of the waiting list for employment at the rail workshops. This proved a unique experience for me as it was the first time I had been confronted with questions from one of the three people on the interview panel whose technical knowledge was probably greater than mine. I was however able to satisfy him on my ability to do the job and was told I would start in No. 5 Shop in the Carriage and Wagon Works till the completion of the current D.M.U. build programme. Upon its completion I would then transfer to the Loco Works or possibly, given my experience, to the Maintenance Shop. Twenty five years later, when the works closed, I had progressed to the role of Chief Foreman of Electrical Maintenance.

However for now I joined the dynamo repair gang in No. 5 Shop of the Carriage and Wagon Works where I was reminded of Woolwich Arsenal both by the buildings and the fact that the large majority of machines in use throughout the different elements of the factory complex ran off a system of shafts and belts much as they had at the start of industrialisation.

Work on the dynamo gang was physically exhausting, the dynamos themselves weighed five to six hundred weight. We had to strip off the end plates, remove the brush gear then lift out the armature which weighed two hundred weight, more often than not, single-handedly. We then had to carry this fifty yards to a makeshift sheet metal booth where the carbon dust was blown out with an airline, the extraction equipment in this booth being at best inadequate and usually all but useless. At the end of the day we would be smothered in carbon dust which would be deeply ingrained in one's skin due to the heavy sweating experienced as a result of the sheer physical effort involved.

This led, one evening, to an entirely unexpected occurrence which caused Joan to be greatly frightened and bought about a situation which, over the years, much to my regret for having been the cause of it, she was never properly able to overcome. I had arrived home, physically shattered, and after dinner had decided I would play with Dawn until her bedtime. I would then soak my aching frame in a nice hot bath. About forty five minutes or so later, having not re-emerged, Joan entered the bathroom curious as to how long I intended to stay in there. When she came in she saw me lying with my feet jammed hard against the end of the bath, my chin on my chest and my nose only just above the water level in water that had clearly grown cold. It was very obvious that I was unconscious. In the five years since we had met she had often seen me in need of glucose but this was the first time she had seen me in that condition as a consequence of my diabetes. Terrified that my head would shift and I could possibly drown she rushed into the living room and dialled 999.

The duty doctor who attended was one from the local practice we had recently joined and he arrived within minutes of her call. Joan had had the presence of mind to leave the door to the flat open before returning to the bathroom to grasp my hair, of which there was plenty in those early days, and pull my head clear of the water. The doctor administered a glucagon injection and helped me out of the bath encasing me in a warm blanket also giving Joan some much needed reassurance. He then admonished me with his oft repeated instruction to "run on green lad" and took his leave!

Aside from her normal monthly situation Joan had, from her early teens, been subject to a niggling ache in her lower abdomen. However she always tended to internalise her problems and concerns rather than discuss them but I could always tell when something was worrying her. Myself, on the other hand, looked at life with a realistic and maybe somewhat blasé attitude of "what will be, will be", especially in relation to my diabetes. Years later Joan was diagnosed with Irritable Bowel Syndrome (IBS) and it is only now that I have realised the amount of pressure my condition put onto her throughout our life together.

About three months after this incident we were lying in bed one night fast asleep when Joan awoke with a start concerned at a gasping, gurgling sound emanating from myself. She reached across to shake my shoulder and discovered I was soaking wet with sweat just pouring off me which had soaked right through everything staining the mattress. This was my first occurrence of night time hypoglycaemia. These night "hypos" occurred approximately once every four years throughout our forty seven years of married life.

The last, and potentially most awkward one, occurred in 1984 when we were crossing Switzerland at night by train on our way to Innsbruck. We occupied a coachette with myself sleeping in the top bunk and Joan in the bunk below. Joan was woken up by moisture dripping onto her face. Balancing on the bar at the edge of her bunk in a swaying carriage she reached up to find me soaked in sweat but not quite unconscious. However I was unable to take a glucose tablet. So, dressed only in her nightgown, Joan set off through the train to get me a sugary drink. I had a hell of a fine wife! When the train arrived at Innsbruck there was a medical team waiting but thanks to the devotion of my wonderful wife their services were unnecessary.

With Dawn nearing her first birthday and the sidecar not yet purchased, one Monday night about two weeks after I had started work at the rail workshops I was riding my Velocette solo and, homeward bound after an E.T.U. meeting. I was riding along a road on the Penhill estate when I noticed a car had mounted the pavement and was buried in the hedge in front of a terrace of houses. A policeman stepped out from behind the car and held up his hand for me to stop. I was travelling quite slowly and merely touched the front brake. Unfortunately this caused the rear wheel to skid to the left thus throwing the bike's full weight against my left leg which I had taken off the footrest. As the bike skidded I came off automatically extending my left hand to break my fall. Now, together with my weight combined with that of the bike, my left hand took the full force of the fall. When the policeman came to my aid and proceeded to swing my left arm back and forth to check if it was O.K. I let out a shrill yell of pain and we both realised that I had broken my collar bone. On my way by ambulance to hospital my main concern was to get a sandwich to avoid having a hypo. As usual I caused the casualty doctor some consternation as my priority was warding off a potential hypo whilst his was obviously to treat my broken collar bone.

This accident certainly made life difficult for me for a few weeks, particularly as my little toddler daughter was a real "daddy's girl" who took great delight in standing on my thighs with her hands on my shoulders rocking back and forth laughing in delight. With Joan seeking to quell our daughter's enthusiasm Dawn could not understand why I was unable to laugh with her!

Over the next couple of weeks, two of our neighbours very kindly retrieved my bike. It transpired that the skid had been caused as a result of mud covering the road from the site of a new junior school that was in the process of construction. This slippery surface had been enhanced by a rain shower about an hour earlier when the car I had seen lodged in the hedge had left the road.

Joan had duly informed my employers what had happened, worried that my sickness absence would possibly lead to my dismissal. This would most certainly have been the case had I still been working in contracting. However, to her immense relief, she had been assured that not only was my job safe but I would be in receipt of sick pay whilst I was off sick which lifted a great weight off her shoulders.

Some three weeks or so later my shoulder was still not up to lifting the armatures so I found myself working on the completion of the Diesel Multiple Unit sets. One Saturday morning, whilst I was sitting on the edge of a pit between the front and rear bogies of the carriage of a three-car set with a blowlamp between my knees preparing to solder two lugs on the ends of cables, I suddenly felt the need to eat my morning sandwich which I did. However, as can sometimes be the case, the action of doing so enhanced rather than diminished the effect of the insulin which had prompted me to eat in the first place. As a consequence I began to lose concentration and found myself slumping forward uncomfortably close to the flame of the blowlamp. My attention was sharply focused when the carriage started to move. I swiftly swung my feet up and out of the pit clear of the blowlamp and rolled backwards. The wheels of the bogie had come less than a yard from severing my legs at the thighs. Some idiot ganger had ordered the unit to be moved without checking that all was clear and safe to do so.

However this incident does serve to demonstrate the need for Type One diabetics to be constantly aware of their physical condition and to ensure they keep their wits about them at all times. We cannot allow ourselves to become complacent but, at the same time, we should not allow ourselves to become unnecessarily paranoid. We just have to use common sense and learn from each experience. If you do, you will enjoy many of these experiences, both good and bad, but all part of the rich pattern of life.

In the spring and summer of 1962 on each Saturday afternoon Joan and I would walk down from Penhill into the central shopping area of Swindon to get our weekly shop. We would have Dawn ensconced in the bassinette her grandparents had bought for us. On these walks we would quite often be stopped by one of my work, E.T.U. or C.P. colleagues, out with their wives on a similar mission. Dawn duly received much fuss and praise that was normally bestowed on new babies and their parents. Joan and I were both deliriously happy and content with our lot in life.

Around this time the Council announced a scheme whereby they proposed to build an estate of houses which would be made available to Council tenants to buy. All that was initially needed was a £25 deposit. The house purchase would include a fixed rate mortgage repayable over twenty five years which averaged around £3,000, dependent upon the type of property, i.e. two or three bedroom or a bungalow. Joan and I discussed joining the scheme but ultimately decided that at that particular moment in time it would not be practicable for us to pursue it.

That spring, although Joan was dubious, I had allowed my name to be put forward as a Communist Party candidate for the Penhill ward in the forth-coming Local Authority elections. Although I was not successful in winning that seat we did however secure a reasonable number of votes and as a consequence of this I became a member of the Tenants Association. Some months later I was elected as Chairman of that organisation.

By the end of the year I found myself working in the No.6 shop of the rail works as one of the one hundred and fifty electricians employed there. We were a real diverse mix of émigrés from all over the U.K. and although many had, not all of these men had necessarily served their time in the factory. We were, without doubt, the most cohesive, organised and best paid group of shop floor workers in the Swindon area at that time.

After a year or so working with this large group of men with monthly shop meetings usually lasting some three or four hours consisting of both left and right wing individuals competing for the role of shop steward, I was probably the most pragmatic amongst us and was duly elected into the role of Shop Chairman with a remit of keeping things fraternal. Although frequently challenged I retained this position until I resigned in 1968 which was both a tactical and strategic decision on my part following a serious disagreement with another Shop Steward.

The winter of 1962/63 was the worst I believe I have ever experienced. The only way to get to work was on foot dressed in full motorcycle gear minus crash helmet but complete with wool-lined boots. I had to trek four miles through knee deep snow both to and from work where I spent the day stripping and rebuilding dynamos. Through the February and March of 1963, I consumed a large number of small bars of fruit and nut chocolate or Mars Bars in those very difficult days. It really was a very tough and difficult period.

In 1963, as a result of the miners' strike, together with a subsequent further dispute in the power industry, the then "Heath" government introduced the three day working week which additionally brought about a strange situation in the local E.T.U. branch. Coupled with this was the added factor of the E.T.U. trial regarding a disputed election result for the national leadership and all these factors, together with a remorseless anti-left press campaign, meant that the right-wing element was becoming increasingly predominant in the Trade Union movement across the nation. However, so far as the E.T.U. was concerned, Swindon bucked this trend. By persistent effort and astute negotiation, the works' sparks managed to alleviate the monetary effects of the reduced working week.

Very conveniently management alleged that a boiler problem was the cause of the lack of warmth throughout the plant but we knew it was just a ruse in their bid to save on costs by cutting down on the heating bills. Strangely however, this so-called boiler problem did not seem to affect the main office block and any workers dallying in corridors and passages in an effort to seek some warmth and respite from the freezing cold shop floor, would constantly be ushered out.

Demands for action were happening all across the works as a result of which the Works Committee decided to call a mass meeting. A dias was duly erected in one of the table roads in the "A" workshop and a loud hailer obtained in order to address the two thousand shop floor workers who would be gathering from a host of different Trade Unions. However on seeing the size of the crowd spread out before them the speakers expected to address the meeting, with the exception of the A.E.U. and E.T.U. conveners, lacked the confidence and the question of chairing the meeting arose. It was known that I had some experience of chairmanship and addressing large groups of people so I was asked if I would consider taking on this task. Having consulted with the respective representatives from all the Unions involved and established their agreement to this proposal I duly found myself facing the largest group of workers I had ever seen.

Aside from one or two jocular remarks about cockney accents and rejoinders of "bloody foreigners" all went well. The two conveners each gave their reports and subsequent recommendations and after I had answered the few questions that were raised I called for a show of hands. The result was very close and I could see that a declaration either way would be exceedingly contentious. Those people on the platform with myself were noticeably worried. Hope-fully, however, I thought there was perhaps one decisive way to make a deci-sion and asked the workers to vote with their feet. I asked for those in support of the recommendation to move to the left of the table road and those oppos-ing it to move to the right. This caused a bit of consternation as there then followed much milling around with men climbing over or around plant, pits, wagons and shunters, etc., but they eventually established themselves safely into two groups. It was now down to me to determine which was the largest, again causing some consternation amongst those on the platform with me.

However, heavily emphasising my position as elected Chair of the meeting, I loudly declared that the recommendation was duly carried. I then instructed people to either return to their respective shops or stay huddled together for warmth! Following an initial silence there was then widespread laughter as the meeting broke up. My colleagues on the platform expressed their gratitude to me for taking control of the meeting and congratulated me on the way I had handled what, in their view, had been a very difficult situation.

Over the next few years, to my great surprise, I was constantly reminded of this episode by the workers across the whole factory who would periodically refer to it whenever our paths crossed during the course of my work. This dispute had lasted for three days and the management were ultimately forced to accept they had been in breach of the legal temperature requirements contained within the Factory Act. Faced with this admission they had no option but to reimburse everyone for loss of pay during that period, albeit only at the basic rate. However, as I was do discover some twenty years later, there had been one group of four workers who had been excluded from this reimbursement. This was something I succeeded in rectifying and will refer to how I achieved this later in my dialogue at a more relevant point.

As a consequence of the power workers' dispute the press launched a campaign against one particular steward in the industry, a man named Charlie Doyle. They sought to make him appear to be the one responsible for the government's imposition of the three day working week. This, together with the change from a left to right wing national leadership of the E.T.U., following the result of a judge's decision with regard to the disputed national election result, led to a situation where a number of union members were either excluded from office or membership, Doyle being one of them.

The Swindon branch protested against this and supported a resolution moved by myself which the branch carried by a subsequently disputed majority. The branch at that time had both a Minute Book which contained recorded details of meetings, and a Branch Secretary who, at the meeting prior to the one at which the resolution had been carried, had dealt with all the correspondence received and sent. The Branch Secretary read out the letter received from Headquarters threatening action against the branch unless it rescinded its resolution. The members were aghast at such an acrimonious decision and questioned how this had come about. A request was then made for the Minutes of the last meeting to be read out and the Minute Secretary, who had been one of the very vociferous few who had opposed the resolution, immediately left the meeting taking the Minute Book with him. This obviously caused some consternation but without the Minute Book to refer to suspicion arose that the recorded entry of my verbal resolution somehow differed to the reality. Other than the copy of the Branch Secretary's letter to Head Office, which I thought accurately covered what I had said, we had no other point of reference to clarify or substantiate our suspicions. We never did discover the truth behind our suspicions and when the branch refused to rescind its resolution the decision was made by the Union Executive to place the branch on suspension for a period of three months.

In the main, the majority of branch members were employed in two key plants, i.e. the rail works and Pressed Steel Fisher, with the remainder employed in contracting, engineering and the M.o.D. I have always contended that as a result of the nature of the trade itself electricians, by inclination, are politically more left than right wing although obviously both are present. By membership however the largest group were from the rail workshops. The composition of the seven members of the Branch Committee reflected this multifaceted employment mix.

At the end of the three month suspension the Executive Council hired a local cinema one Saturday morning and called a meeting to which all members had received a letter of invitation in order, under their aegis, to elect a new committee. The meeting was well attended with some three hundred people in attendance mainly from the rail works and Pressed Steel Fisher. The Executive Council were not pleased when members of the existing committee were re-elected and consequently withheld recognition of the branch for a further six months. Although on a local level funds were still being banked, this caused problems both with other unions locally and also with the employers in some plants as it interfered with national dispute procedures, i.e. in referring disputes to regional or national levels.

During this period I had been transferred from the local carriage and wagon works to the Kenya shunter build programme where it was the norm to work on the shunter from the building and wiring of its control panel to the final acceptance trial of the vehicle. As the sole spark, which was quite challenging, I enjoyed and managed this work right up to the final trial which now, with the advent of blood test meters, would not have been the problem for me that it was in 1963. On one such trial journey outward bound to Stroud I was sitting in the cab of the vehicle and watching the rails on the track as they came towards me. Upon reaching and stopping at Stroud I did a routine urine testing and ate my lunch and having experienced no obvious problems I felt fine.

The return journey however was a different proposition. The view of the rails this time was that of retreating rather than advancing and after a time I began to feel really uncomfortable. Eventually my discomfort was such that I felt it wise to take a glucose tablet but the feeling persisted. Not wishing to take any more glucose I closed my eyes figuring if I was in danger of going into a hypo then I would develop further symptoms. Upon arriving back at the works with the trial successfully completed, I performed another urine test which this time delivered a blue result. I still do not know whether I was in fact on the verge of hypoglycaemia or not and have merely recounted this episode to demonstrate the strange tricks the brain will play when blood sugar begins to drop.

This is merely one of many such incidents I have experienced over the past sixty years but I firmly believe in the principle of taking the minimum amount of glucose necessary to enable you to rationally examine events. Long term hyperglycaemia is the biggest danger to diabetics; this is what can cause loss of sight and limbs, etc.

Within a few days of this incident I was asked to report to the Staff Office. On doing so the Personnel Clerk told me I was required to present myself at a given office number. Intrigued, I asked why I had been summoned and who had called for me. Shaking his head he shrugged his shoulders, apparently it was not a rail works matter.

Therefore I wandered along the passage hoping the number of the office I had been given was located on the ground floor. Eventually, after changing direction at a couple of corners along the passage, I found the office I was looking for and knocked on the door not having a clue as to what awaited me inside. The door was opened by a thickset man whom I estimated to be about six inches shorter than myself. He waved me inside and indicated for me to sit in a chair before a desk behind which, to my amazement, sat Frank Chapple, the recently appointed General Secretary of the E.T.U. following the result of the disputed election for the posts of General Secretary and President. He was later to become "Sir Frank" following his knighthood by Maggie Thathcher's government. I had met him once before although only fleetingly.

With him were two other people who were unknown to myself and from the questions directed at me it soon became evident they were seeking an opportunity to justify and secure the closure of the Swindon branch. I was therefore very guarded in my responses. After some lengthy verbal fencing the suggestion was made that I was possibly endangering my continuance in membership. My response to this was to reach into my jacket pocket, take out my membership card and toss it onto the desk with the words "do with it, what the hell you like, I'll have no difficulty in joining the T&G or N.U.R."! With that I got up and walked out for I knew that nationally the E.T.U. were seeking sole negotiating rights for electricians from the British Rail Board. At that time both the T&G and the N.U.R. were involved in such negotiations. It came as no surprise therefore when, before I had gone ten metres down the corridor, one of the three inquisitors caught up with me and handed back my card with assurances I would hear no more of the matter. Some others were also called before these three but from what I could ascertain were not subjected to similar questioning.

Some months later, and the cause of some media interest, yet another mass meeting was called on another Saturday morning at the previous cinema venue and was, this time, chaired by Les Cannon the General President.

On that Saturday, accompanied by Joan and Dawn on our usual Saturday morning errands, I had walked into town. I did not anticipate that the meeting would be a lengthy one which subsequently proved correct for, with the exception of the former Minute Secretary the previous branch officers, much to the annoyance of those on the platform, were for the third and final time elected unopposed to their previous positions on the committee. The Minute Book however was never returned and the Swindon branch re-opened without further ado.

This outcome was much to Joan's relief for with her propensity to internalise her concerns she had been envisaging all sorts of future employment difficulties in the event that I may be suspended from E.T.U. membership. Despite my repeated assurances however her nature was such that she could not help but worry although, to my mind, unduly. This in turn caused me concern for her health as she was now pregnant with our second child.

That same afternoon we received a much worse shock which caused the pair of us a great deal of alarm. Dawn by now was walking with more confidence and I had been holding her by her reins while Joan and I examined some items on a shop counter. It wasn't until I became aware of the lack of pressure on the grip in my hand and looked down to see the empty harness that I realised she had slipped the reins from her shoulders and wandered off. Searching the shop aisles Joan in desperation we called our daughter's name but all to no avail. Going to the shop door, panic stricken, we looked left and right down the street until we finally caught sight of her some fifty metres away. We hurried up to where she was resolutely trying to extract her hand from the grasp of a middle aged lady proclaiming loudly in an indignant voice "let go you are not my mummy". This lady had seen her leave the shop and having earlier seen the three of us together had caught hold of Dawn to stop her from wandering off. Much relieved we profusely thanked this kind lady and with much protesting from our daughter promptly ensconced her in her pushchair until we returned to Penhill where we allowed her to walk the final half mile.

At that time Dawn had a lovely powder blue linen top coat that Joan had very skilfully made for her. It was with a great deal of pride on my part that I would walk with her, hand in hand, when she was so dressed complete with matching bonnet or beret to the local swings and roundabout which she loved. Many was the Sunday morning I can remember staggering with dizziness as a result of running round in circles to her insistent demands of "faster daddy". Minutes later, clutching my spinning head, my cheeky, rock steady daughter, would announce she wanted to get off and innocently ask "what's wrong daddy, does your head ache"?

Following the tragic accident in which my friends had been killed I had purchased a second hand sidecar and chassis. However Joan found the sidecar to be too claustrophobic but the chassis on the other hand was serviceable. With the cost of a new decent sized seat being beyond our resources I decided to build one myself. Accordingly I prepared a design and duly presented the sketch to Joan for her observations and hopefully approval. Appreciating that the design I had prepared would overcome her claustrophobia in addition to incorporating a separate seat and restraint for Dawn, Joan's only concern was the question of adequate ventilation and the facility to communicate between us. In order to address this I modified my design so that two of the windows could be partially opened. I had subsequently obtained the rental for a garage in the block located in the courtyard below our flat so, gathering together the necessary aluminium, perspex, floorboads and ply I commenced construction which took me a couple of months to complete.

By now Joan's pregnancy was developing to the point where Dawn was asking why her mother's tummy was getting so big. We explained to her that she would be having a baby sister or brother.

With the project now nearing completion, a few weeks later I came up from the garage to the flat to have a break and some lunch. This completed I told Dawn, with whom I had been playing, to stay in the living room and despite her protests I then left and went downstairs believing I had shut the door behind me. As I turned the staircase at the bottom to leave by the rear lobby door heading towards the garage I met the postman who had entered by the front door which was fitted with a delayed action closing mechanism. We exchanged greetings and then went to our respective tasks, me to the garage and him to the upper floors. Some twenty minutes later there was an anxious call to me, hidden from view by the open garage doors, from Joan on the balcony of our flat. She was enquiring whether Dawn was with me. Alarmed

I rushed upstairs, hugged Joan and asked when she had last seen her.

At this point in my writing, recollecting this stressful incident, my shaking legs have forced me to stop and do a blood test which has revealed a blood sugar reading of 14.1. I am certainly not experiencing a hypo but my subconscious mind, recalling my terror at the incident forty eight years ago, has affected my nerves. This only proves to demonstrate the need for Type One diabetics to constantly seek to rationalise one's situation. On this occasion the simple expedient of smoking a roll-up has assisted me to control this episode. Such is the diabetic life!

However, returning to that Saturday afternoon, after two frantic hours of searching, with the help of many of our neighbours and the police, the policewoman who had been left with Joan for comfort took a call on our home telephone from one of her colleagues. It transpired that Dawn had walked the estate until she had recognised the spire of St Peter's church at the end of the road in which Joan's midwife lived. She new this landmark from the numerous journeys in the pushchair she had been with Joan to the midwife. Knowing the midwife lived in the vicinity she had gone down the street knocking on doors demanding to know when her baby was coming.

The baffled neighbours had taken her to the midwife's address where, in answer to her question of where she lived, Dawn had informed her that she lived at number seventy eight down the road, not yet having mastered the pronunciation of the name of our road, i.e. "Downton". Having heard the announcements of a missing child from the loudhailer the police were using outside the amused midwife contacted them and, much to our relief, informed them all was well.

This far outweighed our joy of the successful of another stressful occasion when some months before, upon returning from work, I had found Joan sobbing her heart out. When I asked her what was wrong she told me that she had lost her engagement ring. She was afraid it had slipped off her finger when she had been putting out the rubbish which had been collected that morning. Thinking it highly unlikely I would succeed I did anyway take myself off to the Council tip in an endeavour to find it. However I was forced to return several hours later when, even with the aid of a powerful torch I had borrowed, it had become too dark to see. The search of course proved fruitless and Joan was very much distressed.

A couple of months later, when she picked up her knitting bag one evening to complete a part-knitted garment she had put aside, she suddenly let out a delighted yell of surprise and joy. There at the base of the bag lay her engagement ring. I laughed as I recalled the many hours I had spent hauling aside and tearing open bags of foul smelling rubbish and searching amongst their rotting contents when all the time the thing I was so desperately searching for was sitting comfortably in my wife's knitting bag!

The uncontrollable shaking to which I have already referred had first come to my attention some five years previously. Whilst we were on holiday in Cornwall we visited the Flambards Museum which features a full size realistic diorama of a street scheme from the blitz. I was calmly examining this when suddenly the already dim lighting went down, the siren howled and there was the initial whoosh and then the crump of exploding bombs followed by the crashing sound of falling masonry. I immediately started shaking like the proverbial leaf as the memories came flooding back. I had frequently experienced and lived through this same scenario during the war from the age of two years right up to the two months preceding my seventh birthday. Despite the fact that this had occurred some sixty years earlier I was immediately transported back in time.

However Joan, as a baby in January 1940, had been taken by her mother up to Durham and she had no such buried memories. She consequently looked at me in some alarm suspicious I was close to having a hypo. In the dim lighting of the museum she was unable to clearly see my eyes or forehead but by wiping her palm across my forehead she was reassured by the absence of sweat and reluctantly accepted my reaction was due to my subconscious transmission back to the terrors brought about by the blitz in my early years of life.

In the summer of 1962 we had to go up to London for Colleen and Ron's wedding. Aside from our desire to be there Joan would be acting as Colleen's maid of honour. All went well although to our subsequent amusement Colleen caused our mother some considerable consternation when at the conclusion of the usual panoply of wedding photographs she insisted on having her photograph taken of her in her wedding dress holding her six month old niece. So the requested photograph was taken with Dawn held in Colleen's arms gazing rapturously into her aunt's face.

1963 saw the beginning of the demise of power of the Trades Union movement as a whole which greatly impacted on the aim of the left-wing element of ensuring a greater share of wealth and power for the working class in order to build a fairer society. Once again the electricians were at the forefront.

At the Rules Revision Conference in June of that year, at which I was the delegate from the Swindon branch, the new right wing Executive managed to carry out changes which removed elected area officials and committees replacing them with an appointed area officer. They subsequently did the same with national officers being appointed not elected. Thus, despite vehement opposition, cronyism became the norm as one union after another succumbed to this move away from democracy. In due course this led to a situation which now sees any potential attempt by workers to improve their pay or working conditions frequently becoming subjected to injunctions. From this early example of a Trades Union leader selling out the interests of the membership to the interests of the capitalist system of economics rather than the achievement of socialism, we now find ourselves in a situation where the government of the day, in order to uphold capitalism, is prepared to mortgage the future prosperity of its people to an economic system whose sole aim has always been to subjugate rather than enhance the position of the common man (expression used in its animal sense).

In mid 1964 Joan and I, together with Colleen and Ron, booked a self-catering holiday in a cottage in West Pembrokeshire with Joan, Dawn and I travelling down on the combination bike I had custom built. We all had an enjoyable holiday and our route home took us via Cross Keys which was entered by way of quite a steep hill at the bottom of which was a set of traffic lights. Travelling in front of us was a slow-moving car and as we began the descent I pulled out in preparation of overtaking. However just as I did this a pre-mix concrete lorry turned left at the crossroads below and began its ascent up the hill. I, of course, abandoned the thought of overtaking and swung back in to the left. In order to allow enough room for the lorry to have clear passage I had to manoeuvre such that the wheel of the sidecar mounted the grass verge. This meant I was sitting astride the bike at a thirty degree angle to the horizontal of the road. The sight of this in his rear view mirror alarmed the elderly motorist in the car in front who had likewise stopped at the red light. He got out of the car to enquire if all was OK then stared in horrified disbelief through the front screen of the sidecar at Joan, who was now six months' pregnant, sitting inside with our two year daughter located behind her in her own separate seat. With a hand clasped to his mouth he then fainted. It was now my turn to be concerned but fortunately he recovered quite quickly and his wife assured me all was well. The sight of a woman at that stage of pregnancy apparently often affected him that way although we were none the wiser as to why. Once the lights changed to green we continued on our homeward journey which proved to be uneventful but the episode was, to say the least, a strange experience.

With the birth of our second child now rapidly approaching I found myself working with six other men in the instrument repair room, a unit that was separated from the main shop floor area. One of my colleagues, Ivor Webb, was a judo black belt well able to throw me around as he ably demonstrated on a number of occasions when, for a time, I attended judo classes. However one morning, following an incident in our work area, he paid me an unexpected compliment. The work we were engaged upon was delicate and sedentary, completely different from the more physically demanding tasks of the previous eleven years.

I was no longer cycling to work and this had, to a degree, affected the physical manifestations of the onset of hypoglycaemia. I am now able to adjust to such symptoms, i.e. loss of concentration, self induced prevarication and doubt when making decisions. In the absence of any physical efforts, a reluctance to accept and recognise this could be a pre-warning of an imminent hypo. There were no blood test meters available then and the mental confusion, together with the considerable distance and effort involved in locating and reaching a toilet block to perform a urine test, was beyond my ability once these new and completely unexpected signs had manifested. By that stage I would have reached the point where I would be writhing on the floor, legs and feet kicking out uncontrollably, hands clenched and arms flailing with my spine arching then relaxing and, depending on the depth of the hypo, my head jerking around.

The first of these incidents Ivan had, using his judo skills, attempted to place my flailing limbs in a judo hold to enable one of my other colleagues to spoon feed me with sugar. This I promptly spat out in a subconscious rejection of all things sweet. Ivan told me later that in a hypoglycaemic state I had the strength of ten men which had presented him with his most difficult challenge ever as a judo black belt. He added that I was usually a "pussy cat" but in that state I was worse than a gorilla!

It was following a similar incident some months later that I gave the same advice to my colleagues as I had done to other work colleagues and friends in the past, i.e. in the event of such an incident occurring in the future they should always make sure they stayed well clear of my flailing limbs and, if possible, only approach me from behind. They should then kneel on my arms, between elbow and shoulder, and pinch my nostrils together so that as I opened my mouth for air they could then pour the sweetened liquid into my mouth which I would invariably swallow.

As I slowly adjusted to these new signs of a hypo attack I would normally handle them myself, as I always had. However I was now working as a Work Study Practitioner and the mental prevarication which sometimes arose when writing reports or contemplating alternative methods of performing tasks did occasionally place me and my colleagues in the situation described above. On a few occasions the work's ambulance would be summoned and I would be taken to the casualty department of the local hospital where, sometimes, a glucogen injection or glucose drink would be administered. If I happened to be conscious and thinking straight I would usually resist this as "hyper" rather than hypoglycaemia has always been my main concern, hence the retention of my sight and my feet.

On being discharged from the casualty department I would habitually walk the mile and a half back to work in order to drop my blood sugar levels to the normal blue or green on a urine test. This used to cause the nurse, Kathy, employed by the works in its First Aid Centre some concern. She always told me that whilst I was one of the four people with Type One diabetes employed there who caused her the least problem, my determination not to recognise the condition as a limitation on my activities set me apart and that worried her with regard to my long term prospects.

With the birth of our second child now imminent and knowing that the gate keeper at the Redcliffe Street entrance to the works was not always in attendance I started to park the motorcycle combination on the road outside the gate in readiness for the call that Joan was in labour. Sure enough, the anticipated call came two days before our fourth anniversary, on the 8th October 1964. I climbed the twelve feet high wire fence running alongside the spiked iron entrance gate, which was some fourteen feet high, manipulated myself clear of the spikes arranged on top of the gate, slid down the vertical bars and ran to the combination which hastily took me home. I arrived in plenty of time to be present at the birth of our son who, once clear of his mother, let out a hearty cry. We named him Derek and thankfully his birth had been much easier for Joan than Dawn's although he weighed slightly more.

Both Joan and I were overjoyed. We had the two lovely children we had planned for and nature had granted us what we were told was known locally as a pigeon pair, i.e. a son and daughter. Once the midwife had cleaned him up and presented him wrapped in a shawl to his mother, at her insistence, I hurried into the living room to get Dawn who was delighted to meet her new baby brother. She immediately became very protective of him and protested loudly whenever the midwife or the doctor approached.

As we were to discover over the next three months or so, Derek differed from his sister in one respect. Dawn had been relatively quiet as a baby, sleeping contentedly between feeds. Derek on the other hand was the complete opposite and caused us many a disturbed night as we alternated his feeds, nappy changes, etc., between us. However by the time he reached nine months our curly, blond headed little boy at last settled down into a regular pattern, much to our relief. Our prime night time concern now was the bouncing feet of his two year old sister as she rocked the cot in their bedroom.

With two children we now qualified for a house so saying farewell to our neighbours, who lived in the six flats in our block, we took our leave and moved to an end terrace house in a Close in the valley on Penhill where we lived for three years. Here we had a garden for the children to play in and in which I attempted to grow some vegetables.

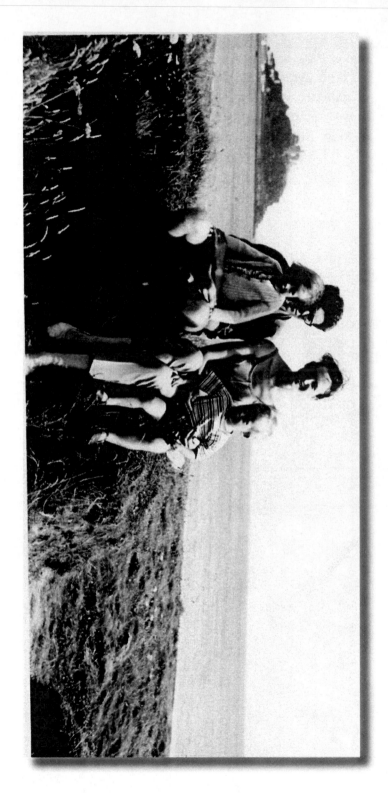

Marazion July '68, Derek aged 2 and Dawn aged 4

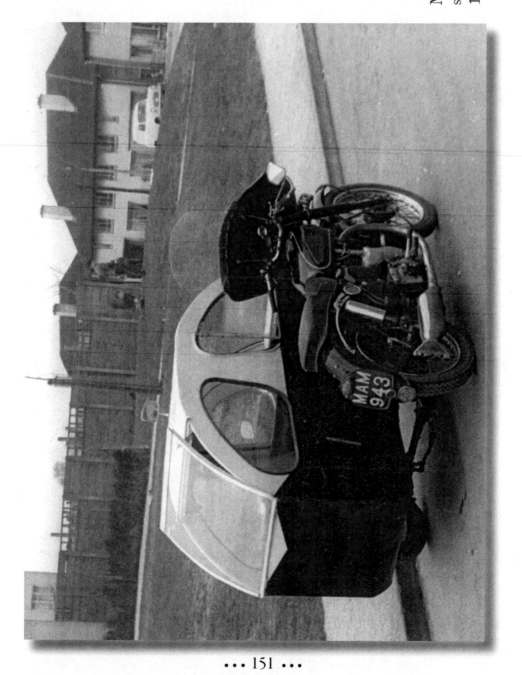

My home-built sidecar, September 1964

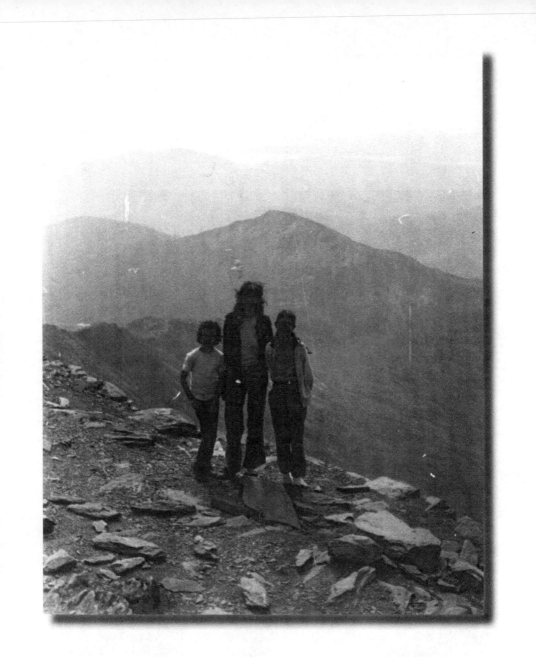

Above and right: Peak of Snowdon achieved Autumn 1971, Dawn aged 9 and Derek aged 7. We walked all the way from the valley below, many sweets consumed by kids and glucose tablets by dad.

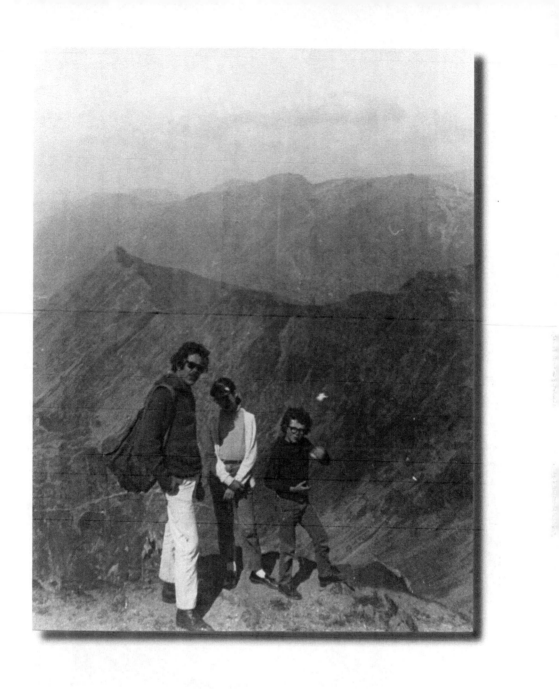

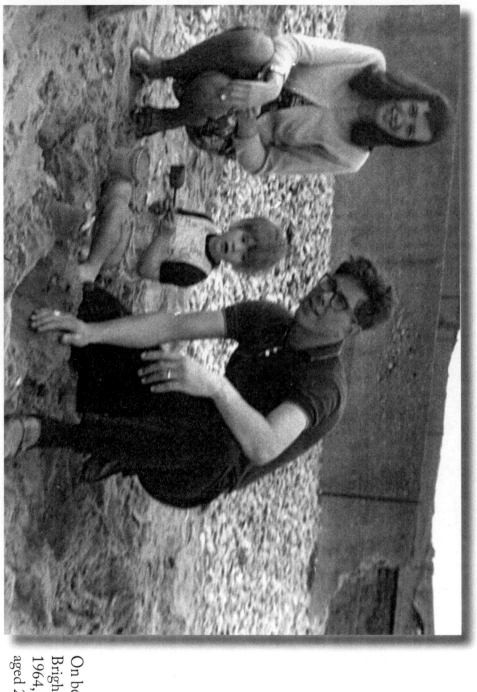

On beach at
Brighton June
1964, Dawn
aged 2

Homeowner and Election to Council

Following much discussion with Joan I then made the second most important decision of my life, the first being when I asked her to marry me. During my working day I would spend some time in making calculations with regard to pursuing the option of taking out a fixed Council mortgage over a twenty five year period with a deposit of just £25. I based my estimations on the likely effects of inflation on Council rents and the subsequent repayments that would fall due over this period. I subsequently decided it was now or never so we went ahead with the purchase of one of the houses the Council were building for sale to its sitting tenants.

My parents were aghast at this decision and Joan's were, to say the least, very dubious and my work colleagues thought I was mad since the Council rate at that time was 6%. However within six years of us taking up this option, i.e. September 1967, the advantage of our situation became clear to all those former sceptics. The raging inflation of the 1970s demonstrated the sense of our gamble and we now owned and occupied a three-bed semi-detached house on one of the most pleasant and desirable, less densely populated estates in the Swindon conurbation.

Soon after this move my mother and father decided to give Joan and I their Ford Consul car as, out of their three children, we were the only ones who did not have one. My father told us he had decided it was cheaper for them to hire a car for their occasional weekends away but we firmly believed the true reason was their fear of our perceived vulnerability in using our motorbike combination. Thus it was that I learned to drive a car and very soon after that we took up camping.

Prior to our move to Covingham however there had been two incidents which had caused Joan some alarm. The first of these occurred one Sunday afternoon. As was my habit at that time, I had spent the morning fishing. The children had gotten used to this and when they asked Joan where I was she would always give the same response – "oh he's gone fishing". On this particular occasion I had landed a seven pound pike which, on a friend's recommendation, I decided to eat. I therefore took it home with me wrapped inside a wet towel and placed it in the Belfast sink in the kitchen. I left it there while I went into the shed to deposit my fishing gear and change my clothes. Suddenly there was a blood curdling scream upon which I rushed back into the kitchen to be confronted by a white faced Joan who, pointing at the sink asked "what is that?" as she nervously edged away. Although the pike was constrained by the sides of the sink it was thrashing about, flexing its spine and raising its head and tail. I quickly lifted it out of the sink and speedily despatched it by a swift blow to the head. The fish proved to be very tasty indeed and Joan sewed two of its teeth into my fishing hat as a memento. Other than the occasional eel, that pike was the only freshwater fish I ever ate from the many I subsequently caught over the years.

The second incident was even more frightening for Joan. By now Dawn was big enough to open the rear garden gate and one day, seeing one of her play-school friends near the garages with her father, who also owned a combination motorcycle, she opened the gate and went out to join them. Trotting behind, Derek had followed her down the garden and unfortunately had his hand on the gatepost as she shut the gate. His screams brought Joan and the father of Dawn's little friend running to him in a panicked response. They discovered that the tip of one of his fingers had been severed. Joan wrapped his hand in a cloth, retrieved the severed finger tip and was rushed to A&E by a kind neighbour where they were able to re-attach it. Fortunately, in later years, this accident did not hinder Derek's flexibility or manoeuvrability in his subsequent trade as a tool maker. To the intense pride of myself and his mother he went on to graduate with a B.S.C. degree in engineering and production management.

Derek had one other health-type problem and that was a lazy eye, which was a genetic fault apparently inherited from my side of the family. When this was not overcome by blocking off the eye it was ultimately corrected following an operation just after his fourth birthday.

One Sunday afternoon we all examined the different types of houses that were then being built on the second phase of development in Covingham. Joan was not really enthusiastic about any of the designs. We still had a copy of the drawing of the type we had both admired on the first phase but were disappointed to find it had been deleted from the second phase. I pointed out to Joan, who had never had to do so, that she lacked the ability of being able to transcribe a floor plan drawing in her mind into a vision of what the finished article would look like. As this was a natural requirement of my trade I had no trouble in doing so. I further pointed out to her that one of my dynamo bench colleagues did occupy the Colonial design type of house we were interested in so maybe it would be a good idea for us to visit and ask his wife, Betty, if she could show us round their home. Although initially scepti--cal Joan eventually agreed to this.

After Betty had dutifully taken Joan on a tour of her home Joan determined that nothing else we had seen so far could compare and consequently she would not be happy with any other type of house. So, knowing it was a condition of sale that in the event the purchaser ultimately decided to sell then it had to be back to the Council, I went ahead and entered our name onto the list for the next available Colonial style house. One eventually became available in September 1967. The house was now three years old and was on the market for a price of £3,600. This represented a thirteen percent increase on its original cost and the mortgage was two percent higher than that available three years earlier. However as this type of house had not been available then I thought it was worth the risk and now, some forty two years later, I knew I had been right.

A couple of years later as the children would soon both be at school, Joan decided she would apply to the Post Office for an evening job as a telephone operator. This would both supplement the family's income and also provide her with some social contact with other women. Soon after she started her job a dramatic and potentially dangerous incident occurred. This particular evening the four of us had, as usual, finished our evening meal and I together with the children had waved Joan off to work at 6.45 p.m. as she left for her 7.00 p.m. start time. After I had washed up I was indulging the children in our usual "rough and tumble" play session before they went to bed although maybe more boisterously than usual. On this occasion my digestion and the insulin I had injected before our meal was somewhat slower than usual in taking effect. Myself and the children were having a lot of fun and I can remember I was crawling along the living room floor and found myself very near to the bottom glazed door which led to the small entrance lobby. It was at that point that the insulin asserted itself and my back arched in response. My legs jerked straight out behind me and my head was thrown forward with such force that it smashed through the glass. Had my back arched again I would either have cut my throat or the back of my neck. My six year old daughter knew immediately what was wrong and bravely took command of the situation. Grabbing my hair to hold my head up she instructed me to move backwards, telling me I needed some sugar. I had sufficient sense to obey and having accomplished this she then told me to turn onto my back. She then told her four year old brother to sit on my chest and hold my nose following which she went into the kitchen. I could hear a stool being moved and the noise of a tap running and Dawn re-appeared saying "two spoons of sugar daddy, drink". Some ten minutes later, having recovered, I sat there and heard my daughter asking to speak to Joan Huzzey on the telephone after dialing 100. She described what had happed to her mother and asked her if she had done the right thing. I sat there stunned in amazement at my daughter's command of the situation but full of great pride at such an achievement in one so young. This was to be the first of many such occasions when I had to rely on my children to administer glucose albeit never again in such dire circumstances.

There was a similar incident some two years later and one which the children used to regularly relay to their friends claiming that no-one could clear a station platform as quickly as their daddy. It happened on the platform of the Northern Line at the Oval. We had walked to the station after visiting their maternal grandparents and arrived to find a very crowded platform. By that time my gait was becoming extremely slow and as there was a chocolate dispensing machine on the wall I decided to buy a treat that was usually denied me. The machine, however, decided otherwise. After feeding it with five coins and thumping it in exasperation it still withheld the desired chocolate bar. Not understanding my condition people had edged away when I had first approached the chocolate machine. By now, however, my arms and legs were flailing and as if by some hidden command the platform suddenly cleared although no train had as yet arrived. This left Joan, I and the children desperately trying to get some chocolate from the machine which was still stubbornly refusing to give it up. At the appearance of a West Indian station attendant Joan hurriedly explained our predicament and he beckoned for us to follow him. Leading us further down the platform he unlocked a door and ushered us into a room reappearing a few minutes later with cups of tea for myself and Joan and glasses of milk for the children. Out of the myriad of people on the platform that day, this man was the only one to display any concern and assistance, on top of which he insisted in reimbursing me with the half crown ($12^1/_2$ p) I had lost in the chocolate machine.

Around this time Joan had formed a friendship with one of her older work colleagues, a lady named Doreen. She and her husband, Gordan, had recently purchased a Volkswagon Caravanette and in the absence of any grandchildren of their own had offered us the loan of the tent they had used previously so that we, as a family, could accompany them on a weekend break to the Forest of Dean. The children were of course eager to go so one Friday evening we all set off. We emerged from our first night under canvass on the following Saturday morning to a beautiful sunny day. Rubbing their still sleep filled eyes the children both declared that their beds had been a bit hard and they had heard strange snuffling noises during the night which we later discovered was nothing more than a hedgehog. However we all enjoyed the experience.

Earlier that same year we had all spent an enjoyable two weeks' holiday at Marazion in Cornwall with Colleen, Ron and their first child, Mark, in a converted G.W.R. Pulman Coach, known as a "camping coach". The three cousins had thoroughly enjoyed themselves, particularly waving to the train drivers as they blew their hooters at us from the adjacent working track as their trains pulled slowly into Penzance. Each evening the three of them could be found clamouring to be taken to the platform off of which the camping coach was parked. These holiday coaches could be booked through the Rail Staff Association and demand for them was intense and success in booking them two years in succession was virtually impossible.

Therefore, following our enjoyable break in the Forest of Dean, we decided to buy a second-hand frame tent in good condition. On our first attempt at camping we set off after lunch one day on an exploratory walk through the forest. Derek was now four years old and managed to toddle three miles unassisted before becoming too tired to walk any further so accepting a welcome ride on his father's shoulders. Meanwhile his six year old sister would stop periodically to pick a flower which she would place between the pages of a notebook that Doreen had given to her. Dawn happily completed our six mile trek having extracted a promise from me to make her a flower press. This I duly did before our next camping trip.

We had succeeded in purchasing a Marechal frame tent from a couple who were upgrading to a caravan. Following a family conference the children had eagerly supported the idea of staying on a farm rather than more organised camp sites. Having re-weather proofed the tent we gradually, over the years, acquired all the necessary equipment we needed to allow us to camp on just basic sites. The only outside requirement we needed was a reliable water source. Over the course of the next ten years we visited and walked in all the National Parks and toured Scotland twice.

Following a three week stay on Exmoor, where the children had climbed a hill and looked down on a holiday camp in Minehead below, we decided we would somehow find the financial resources to take them there for a week's holiday, intrigued to see if they preferred that to camping. At the end of that week however they announced that whilst they had enjoyed themselves they really did prefer camping. With this established we decided to upgrade to a trailer tent, a few of which we had much admired whilst attending Camping Club meetings.

Joan had by now learned to drive but the division of labour between us was established. I did the driving and erecting the tent, route planning for walks, etc., and she did the cooking and packing. The children's tasks were to obtain water and take charge of the proper disposal of rubbish. As a family we resolutely observed the responsibility of "leaving only footprints behind" which, between the four of us over the course of those ten years, must have been in the millions.

Of course my diabetes always determined that we carried sufficient food when out walking and Joan perfected a wonderful fruit cake which she cooked in a loaf tin. Three or four of these cakes would always accompany us on a week away and the four of us would eagerly eat a thick slice of it around 3.00 p.m. whenever we were out on a walk.

Before their tenth birthday the children walked up the slopes of Snowdon, continuously harassing their dad to catch up. Unhindered by her smoking habit Joan kept pace but hampered as I was by the need to stop and take a glucose tablet every so often, meant I was the last to reach the summit, heart pounding. Once there Joan and I proudly photographed each other with the children.

The only really serious incident with the diabetes occurred some three years earlier when, on a very wet and windy weekend, we had been at a Camping Club anniversary meeting on a farm just outside Calne. The Yetties, a popular west country folk group of the time, had been booked to host a barn dance which was taking place in a marquee on the Saturday evening. The ground in the marquee had been strewn with straw and bales placed strategically around for the audience to sit on. Like most everyone else, we wore Wellingtons as our walking boots would easily have been topped by the mud. We all had a lovely evening and the children consumed a fair amount of fizzy drinks. Joan enjoyed a couple of vodka and orange drinks which were available from the bar counter that had been set up and I satisfied myself with a couple of pints of my own home brew. After three hours of singing and stomping up and down in square dances with our fellow campers, we tiredly and gingerly made our way back through the mud to our trailer tent arriving back around midnight.

About two and a half hours later Joan woke up in alarm to find me sweating profusely. She tried unsuccessfully to rouse me and I was still unresponsive some ten minutes later even after she had pinched my nostrils and poured sweet warm water down my throat. I was now apparently unconscious so Joan hastily pulled on a sweater and trousers and rushed out to summon the meet's steward to contact a doctor. Obviously mobile telephones had not been invented then so the steward in his turn had to knock up the farmer in order to use the house land line. Upon seeing me the doctor immediately sent for an ambulance which arrived some fifteen minutes later. This vehicle had to drive onto the site in order to pick me up but within a matter of only fifty yards from the field entrance it sank axle deep into the mud and could go neither forwards or backwards. This left the ambulance crew with no option but to summon a second ambulance with strict instructions not to drive onto the camp site.

By now Joan was growing really alarmed but with the constant reassurances of the ambulance crew watched as I was carried off site on a stretcher and placed in the second ambulance. The sugared drink she had given to me earlier eventually brought me back to consciousness just as the ambulance pulled into the A&E Department at Swindon's Princess Margaret Hospital and despite my protestations the ambulance crew insisted I sit in a wheelchair to be taken inside.

This incident took place before Joan had mastered the art of driving and after I had drunk a glucose draft, at the insistence of the attending medic, I protested that I should be taken back to Calne as it was down to me to collect my family and drive them home. They, quite rightly of course, pointed out that an ambulance was not a taxi. I in turn adamantly declined to eat breakfast or take any insulin at the hospital. I further pointed out that having lived with diabetes now for more than fifteen years I knew what I was doing. A compromise was reached, however, when a nurse who lived near Calne and was about to finish her shift offered to drop me off near the camp site. I gratefully accepted her kind offer and around 9.00 a.m. on a bright and warm Sunday morning I returned to the camp site. As I wished my bemused fellow campers a good morning it was with some embarrassment that I revealed to them it was myself who had been the cause of their animated discussions of the previous night's events.

Later that day, at 12.00 noon, when attending the habitual coffee morning gathering at Club meets, I apologised for disturbing everyone's previous night's sleep and for causing so much inconvenience, giving them a brief resume of its cause for future reference. They in turn reassured me they would have ensured that Joan and the children would have been taken safely home had I not returned. What is more the farmer had used his tractor to free the ambulance that had first arrived from its mud logged predicament. He had further reassured everyone that the same assistance would be provided to anyone else who needed it. To a degree, this comment was directed primarily at Joan and myself since, with the demise of the Consul, I was now driving a Renault 4 which only had a 950cc engine. However, like the Citreon 2CV, it had been designed as a utility vehicle to be used by French farmers and to the great surprise of many of our fellow campers we were able to drive off that sodden site unaided. The power to weight ratio of our unit made it somewhat easier to drive than the Land Rovers attached to the caravans. However, although both vehicle types had been designed with farmers in mind, the Renault's front wheel drive design made it much more manoeuvrable in these types of conditions.

The rig did, however, subsequently prove to have two faults, the first revealed itself that autumn when, on a wet evening I was driving through Cardiff on the homeward journey from a weekend on the Gower Coast and on nearing a pedestrian who was crossing the road I applied the brakes. Even though I had the brake pedal fully depressed the weight of the trailer tent, which was not fitted with brakes, pushed the car forward. Fortunately however it stopped just short of the crossing.

The trailer's manufacturer, Concraft, assured me that brakes could not be fitted to it but I was not convinced. As the wheel centres were the same as those on the Mini I purchased two scrap brake drums and a new towing hitch for the trailer. Three months later I drove the whole thing down to the Concraft plant to prove them wrong. The manufacturer was suitably intrigued and congratulated me on what I had achieved. Whether or not they ever adopted my modification I do not know or indeed even if this manufacturer is still in existence.

As with most other things, holidays have, with the new consumer orientated society, changed considerably in the past thirty years. My grandchildren find it incomprehensible that the only entertainment their parents had in the car was to sing along with the "Spinners" or the "Dubliners" to sea shanties on a portable twelve volt single speaker tape player.

The second fault in our Renault revealed itself the following year. After spending a week in the Lake District camped alongside Bassenthwaite Lake and walking up Skiddaw Great Gable and other peaks, we decided to continue up into Scotland. As we left the site, however, an amusing incident occurred. The weather that week had been quite good, apart from the occasional heavy shower, the last of which had occurred on the night prior to us moving out. The morning of our departure was bright and warm and I, as usual, was wearing shorts. In view of the fact that it was a decent day Joan decided she would do the same. The rainfall of the previous night had left the site very wet and pulling away was proving quite difficult so Joan climbed out and went to the back of the car to push to allow the rear wheels to gain traction. She was on the receiving end of a fair amount of spray before the front wheels finally bit and the unit jerked forward. Once moving she hurried back inside and her beautiful legs soon dried to a light brown hue. With a grin and a wink at the children in the back seat we kept quite about it.

We crossed the border at Gretna Green and the children asked if we could stop for ice creams which I agreed to do when we got to the next village. When we found a shop with an ice cream sign Joan got out to buy them and as she got back in she indignantly proclaimed "you rotten lot, you might have told me! I heard two women in there saying 'aren't southerners strange, fancy wearing stockings with shorts and scholls"!

A couple of days later, as I changed gear to turn left to see Eilean Dunoon Castle at Dornie, I lost drive and we had to push the whole rig onto a small site. Although the engine was running I could not engage the engine drive which to me suggested that the clutch had gone. When I lifted the bonnet to investigate I discovered that the clutch cable had pulled out from the nipple which connected the cable to the clutch itself. So the next morning, having removed the cable, I hitched a lift to Kyle of Lochalsh and caught the ferry to Skye which was where the nearest garage was located. Needless to say they did not have any spare cables and told me the nearest Renault agent was at Inverness on the opposite side of the country. They could order one by post but it would take at least a week to arrive. However they could try to re-solder the nipple and although I was sceptical I agreed it was worth a try. From my own soldering experience I was not impressed with their mechanic as I watched him use the welding torch.

However on completion I made my way back to the ferry and so across to Dornie where I re-fitted the cable and fired up the engine in an attempt to get it to engage. As I had suspected this met with no success and the re-soldered nipple had failed to hold. In despair and at Joan's suggestion I went off for a pint. I was soon engaged in conversation with a couple of local men who had seen us arrive the previous day and had watched me working on the car. They asked what the problem was and during my explanation I have to admit that I may have made some uncomplimentary comment about the Scots being great with riveting guns but no bloody good at soldering. As it turned out these men worked for a haulage outfit and kindly offered me the use of their workshop if I wanted to try to fix it myself. Thanking them I borrowed a blow lamp, vice and solder and set about trying to re-solder the nipple in place and then reassemble it to the car. Success!!

So the following morning we all resumed our journey north. At one stage, some ten miles after leaving Dornie, we caught up with a Land Rover in the back of which I was intrigued to see what I assumed to be two large sacks of carrots which I pointed out to the children. As we were generally running downhill I overtook this vehicle and the children, who were looking through the rear window, noticed a lad around their age sitting next to the driver.

Over the next few miles the glorious scenery was, for the most part, ignored by them as they opened up an exchange with this lad by the use of various hand gestures, etc.

All was going well until, on a particularly steep hill between Strathcarron and Achnasheen as I changed down, the clutch cable again gave out and I pulled over to the side of the road in helpless despair. As previously mentioned, this was the second fault with the Renault. We were miles from any habitation and there were very few other vehicles on the road. None of us could remember seeing a telephone box anywhere since leaving Dornie some twenty miles back. Therefore I was tremendously relieved when, with a toot on the horn, the Land Rover we had overtaken earlier pulled in about one hundred yards in front of us. Getting out, the driver came over to us and asked what was wrong. I explained our predicament informing him that the nearest Renault agent was located in Inverness to which he replied that that was his destination. He then said that if I was prepared to take the risk he would happily tow us across although neither of us had a solid tow bar. I gratefully accepted his offer and in some trepidation we set off, the three vehicles connected only by a rope in which fashion we traversed from one side of Scotland to the other on just a single track road dotted here and there with passing spaces.

There were a few occasions en route when our little convoy consisting of the Land Rover pulling our Renault and trailer tent had to carefully squeeze into a small layby to allow vehicles travelling in the opposite direction to pass. However, some hours later our saviour finally dropped us off on the forecourt in front of the Renault agent. He indignantly refused my offer to buy his son some sweets who, by now, had struck up quite a firm friendship with Dawn and Derek. He pointed out that in the west of Scotland it was the established rule that you helped each other out when the need arose. All that was required in return was a simple thank you which I had already proffered.

In stunned surprise I was really impressed when he then asked to be excused as he had to hurry off to deliver the two sacks of prawns, I had mistakenly assumed were carrots, before he missed the market. I was quite speechless at the realisation that this kind man had endangered his chance of selling his load in order to help us. I was left wondering how on earth the Scottish people had ever earned the reputation of being dour and reputedly tight with money. That perception was perhaps one of the greatest misconceptions I have ever encountered either then, previously or on subsequent visits to that scenically glorious country. I can honestly say that I have never met with anything other than the exact opposite of these two alleged traits.

In 1968 the Unions had signed an agreement with the management of British Rail Engineering Ltd to introduce a productivity scheme based on the introduction of work study. The electricians' shop committee, of which I was Chairman, had followed the lead given by the senior steward that we should reject its introduction out of hand. I had argued that we should initially find out what the scheme entailed and with that in mind had applied to go on a course at the Union college in Esher. So a few weeks later I duly presented myself at Esher together with about twenty five other representatives from other rail workshops around the country.

I was sharing a room with a Guyanese man who lived in Lewisham and worked for London Transport. We two, being the only ones with any experience of the London social scene, were asked by a number of the others if we would take them round the West End. This we did one evening and they were not impressed, particularly by the price of a pint!

When we got back to the college I did not actually get into my bed as lying horizontal after three or four pints usually made sleep difficult. I therefore decided to doze off in an armchair. After two or three hours my roommate became concerned by the strange snuffling noises I was emanating and failing to rouse me went off in search of assistance. He returned with Roy Sanderson, one of the lecturers, who took one look at me and immediately recognised the signs of a hypo for the Type One diabetic as his wife also had this condition.[6]

This incident happened on the last night of the course and I now found myself in Kingston Hospital. Knowing Joan would be expecting me home, Roy telephoned her to explain what had happened, assuring her that everything would be O.K. Having been in the same position himself, with regard

6   Observant readers will recall the incident in hospital with Brian when I was originally diagnosed and will note this describes his tragic circumstances. The third example of nocturnal hypoglycaemia associated with alcohol, either beer, spirits or wine, has the unfortunate propensity to cause catastrophic falls in blood sugar, invariably at the most difficult time when one is sleeping. Therefore the loss of consciousness occurs with no perceptible indication to the diabetic victim themselves. This is very dangerous and the danger can be enhanced if the drinking of alcohol is also associated with simultaneous exercise, i.e. walking, dancing or general exuberant behaviour.

The lesson here is if going for a drink ensure you also have adequate carbohydrate intake, particularly if any exercise will be involved. I am, and never have been, either teetotal or a killjoy but the key, as always, is to be sensible. Do not drink to excess, use your common sense and be aware of the possible consequences. Additionally also make sure that those around you are also aware of the ramifications of mixing too much alcohol with exercise. Remember that too much alcoholic for the diabetic can prove fatal, particularly to Type One diabetics. Whilst drink is not the sole cause of nocturnal hypoglycaemia it must never be forgotten that it can lead to it, therefore only drink in moderation.

to his wife, he knew exactly how Joan would be feeling. He told her that he would collect me from the hospital himself which he did at around midday.

Back at the college later that afternoon Lou Britz, one of those who had accompanied Frank Chapple at my earlier inquisition in Swindon, took me aside and told me that if I changed my allegiance and attitude as far as the leadership was concerned then a National Officer job may be available to me. I responded that I firmly believed in the election process not direct appointment to which he shrugged and said "when are you lot going to learn?"

I telephoned Joan to let her know that I was alright and that I would be home in time for dinner. After thanking Roy and with a parting word to the others on the course I then set off for home. Later that evening, after recounting the day's events, I promised a worried Joan that I would withdraw from active participation in politics and Union events until after the children were well settled into senior school. This decision was also influenced by two other factors.

Firstly, further convinced by what I had learned on the Union course with regard to the techniques on which the rail scheme would be based I did the following. With no intention of doing anything other than treating it as a training opportunity I applied for the post of Work Study Engineer in the knowledge that a shop policy had been adopted which allowed a shop floor spark to perform a temporary staff role as an Inspector or Foreman, for example, for a three month period at the end of which, if they felt they were unsuited to it or were found to be unsuitable, they could then return to their shop floor post. Applicants were required to take and pass an eight week training course before acceptance to the post. I therefore felt this would enable me to become proficient to a degree, absorb knowledge and, I assumed, return to the shop floor within the three month period as stipulated.

So together with another man from the instrument room and two other men from the factory, I took the course. This was broken down into two, four week blocks and at the end of the first block I told the other three of my intention to return to the shop floor. They thought I was off my head as staff status was considered to have many advantages even though the post to which we may be appointed, although guaranteed, was only marginally better paid and I was already covered by sick pay. However other than the odd day here and there and the time when I broke my collar bone or the two weeks I had taken off after contracting chicken pox from the children, I had never had cause to take sickness absence in the twenty five years I worked there.

However my plan was blown out of the water when, on passing the course and reporting to the shop floor, I announced my intention of rejecting the job to be told that the temporary staff release policy had been rescinded. Sympathetic colleagues informed me of their suspicions that this decision, together with a change in the composition of the Shop Committee, had been deliberately engineered to prevent my return to the shop floor.

Thus it was that I found myself trapped in a lethargic and sedentary existence which I abhorred. In that first year working in the office it was all too frequently the case that we had very little to occupy us so in order to keep myself intellectually occupied I completed a number of postal courses set by Oxford's Ruskin College on Europe's Struggle for Unity, Economics and Industrial Psychology and Work Study for Trades Unionists. As a result of the content and quality of my submissions on these courses I had been urged to submit an application to become a student at the University. However as the sole bread winner at that time and not wishing to spend my nights away from my family I declined the offer.

Around this time the diabetes occasionally gave me and my colleagues, when trying to render assistance, problems as the physical manifestation of the onset of a hypo gave way to more pronounced mental indications which caused confusion. Adjustment to these new symptoms was difficult until the introduction of blood test meters in the mid 1970s.

Throughout this period I established a reputation in the office of always projecting the interests of the men on the shop floor. As a consequence, on a number of occasions, I found myself in conflict with my Departmental Head when I refused point blank to amend reports I had submitted for the attention of the Works Manager. This situation came to a head one day when I was summoned to the office of the Works Manager who asked me to explain my report which was causing him some concern. My explanation however proved to be at odds with its content so passing me the report he asked me to explain further. A quick examination of the document confirmed my suspicions. The document before him was not the report I had originally submitted but the amended version I had refused to endorse. I pointed this fact out to him together with an explanation of the potential problems which would arise if the amended report was adopted which he confirmed was the reason for his concern.

The Works Manager subsequently informed the Head of the Work Study Department that henceforth all reports I was asked to submit should go directly to him. What was more I would now be seconded to a team charged with the re-organisation of the whole factory area to a space that was fifty percent smaller than it currently occupied yet still maintaining the diversity and levels of output then being achieved.

Before beginning this however, together with another colleague, I was assigned one further investigation and that was the scrap recovery activity. This was carried out at the far perimeter of the factory where three men worked in absolutely appalling conditions in one of the most dangerous and dilapidated buildings in the works. These three men had, for years, but to no avail, continually raised matters of concern with regard to Health and Safety issues. However their main grievance was against both the Works Committee and Management because, unlike all the other shop floor workers, they had not received the three days' pay everyone else had following the cold weather dispute some years earlier. This decision was based on the grounds that because the nature of their work meant they were always exposed to the full force of the elements then they did not qualify for this payment.

From my days as a spark in the building industry I fully appreciated the men's situation with regard to their working location. Given that our investigation took place in late February my colleague also very quickly appreciated their predicament, particularly in the absence of any sheltered or enclosed space in which we could work.

On completion of our survey my colleague suggested that I should write the report as he felt I could do so more cogently than he could so I happily agreed. Having subsequently submitted the completed report to the Department Head, he threw up his hands in horror. Not only was it highly critical of the working environment but, in view of the recovery of brass, copper, etc., and refurbishable components, it also meant that, in economic terms, the labour return for those three men was amongst the highest in the works. We therefore recommended they be paid an average of the bonus earned throughout the works, plus the missing three days cold weather payment and the provision of heated accommodation for relaxation periods. The Department Head asked that the report be toned down which I refused to do adding that if this was done without our agreement then the original would be leaked to the Works Committee which it subsequently was.

Some months later the three men concerned delightedly informed us they had received the three days' pay for the period in question and had also been provided with a shed in which to take their tea breaks. Additionally, they were now also receiving a bonus. However, as it turned out, they were subsequently only to receive these things which had been denied them, for the next five years or so as the works finally closed in 1986. I must admit, following the successful re-organisation exercise, it gave me a great deal of satisfaction that, having refused to tone down my report, I managed to achieve justice for these men.

After the unfortunate demise of one of my former electrical colleagues and following my desire to return to my trade, I moved sideways and become and Electrical Quality Control Inspector. Later on and with the support of the Chief Draughtsman, Inspector and also Personnel, I was appointed as Chief Electrical Maintenance Foreman. This latter post went against the wishes of the Works Engineer with whom I had previously crossed swords and was also destined to do so again.

By now, in the mid 1970s, the children had both entered senior school and during that time my only political and Trade Union roles had been to act as a shadow staff representative. I had also canvassed on behalf of the local Labour Party branch at both local and parliamentary elections and served as a Labour nominee on the Parish Council.

In 1980 however, following the defeat of the Labour Government in 1979 and the loss of the Swindon parliamentary seat to the Tories, the Swindon Labour Party set out to wrest control of the Borough Council from the Conservatives who had had to introduce a supplementary rate in order to overcome incompetence in the setting of the previous year's budget. This of course did not go down at all well with the people of the borough.

Although I was not a member at that time, other than by Trades Union affiliation, I was a reasonably frequent attendee at local branch meetings where one evening in early 1980, to my surprise, I was asked to stand as the Labour Party candidate for the Covingham ward in the local Council elections.

Joan raised no objections to this and indeed the idea amused her as one of her colleagues with whom she worked at the telephone exchange and who was also a reasonably close neighbour of ours, was the wife of the sitting Tory Councillor. However, even though this lady was from the same working class people as ourselves, Joan contended that she was disinclined to accept this fact as she tended to harbour all sorts of airs and graces purely on the strength of her husband being a Councillor. Joan very much looked forward to her reaction when she became aware that I may be standing as his political opponent which was, however, by no means guaranteed.

Firstly, it was a Labour Party rule that one had to be an individual member for a minimum of three months prior to standing as a Party candidate, which I was not. Secondly, the Swindon Labour Party G.M.C. was strongly under the influence of a Trotskyite entireties group which, by the mid 1980s, had evolved into the so-called militant tendency. They were well aware of my previous Communist Party affiliations, which I allowed to expire after Czechoslovakia in 1968, so it was unlikely they would support my nomination. However Covingham came under the auspices of the Devizes Constituency

G.M.C. who, at the insistence of the Lower Stratton branch which covered Covingham, sought a dispensation from the Party N.E.C. to allow my name to go forward. This was granted and therefore, to the annoyance of the clique on the Swindon G.M.C. and despite their endeavours to overturn it, I became the confirmed candidate.

Following quite a tight campaign and a host of recounts on the night following the 1980 local elections I became the sixth new Labour Councillor to be elected that night having defeated the sitting member by just seven votes which was the closest result of the evening. Labour had, as a result, taken control of Thamesdown Borough Council, the name adopted following Local Government re-organisation in 1974.

The following evening having, during the morning attended a brief seminar on Local Government after being sworn in on the night of the count, I attended my first group meeting and the lack of control or any form of protocol left me absolutely astounded and appalled. The meeting started at 7.00 p.m. and some two and a half hours were taken up solely with arguments as to whether the meeting had achieved a quorum. This was due to the fact that one member had failed to turn up, not even tendering an apology for absence, and one or two individuals were endeavouring to delay the election of the Chair of Housing until the missing member was in attendance.

The appointments to committees and the election of all other Chairs proceeded without any problems. The election of Vice Chairs however exposed a very obvious split between those whose membership duration was in the order of three to five years and the more senior element.

The six newly elected Councillors looked on puzzled until I pointed out that although new to Local Government I did have some experience in Trade Union affairs and I was eager to know what policies and objectives we wished to pursue and how and when we intended to achieve them as that was what I had assumed the meeting was here to address. I further pointed out that from what I had seen so far I had come to the conclusion that this meeting amounted to nothing more than a primary school class and unless we got down to real issues, like the fact that the Tories' supplementary rate would clearly result in serious financial problems, then I for one was going home at 10.30 p.m. This drew a number of muffled "here, here's" from those present.

The following morning, in order to familiarise myself with their respective areas of responsibility, I attended the Council offices to meet the Chief Officers of the two committees onto which I had expressed a desire to serve, i.e Arts & Recreation and Housing. Whilst there I came across the member who had, at the previous evening's meeting, been seeking to delay the proceedings. This was a man with whom I was familiar following a dispute in one of the local factories where he was an A.E.U. steward. I suggested to him that it would be appropriate to adopt a procedure familiar to us both from our respective Trade Union experience and organise a meeting of like minded individuals at a location away from the Civic Offices with a view to establishing objectives on which we were agreed and the means of achieving them. He accepted this was a good idea and volunteered to arrange such a meeting after we had agreed who we thought it most appropriate to approach in this regard.

This meeting took place two weeks later at a hotel on the outskirts of the town with a sixty percent group attendance in terms of length of Council service which was predominantly the junior element of the group. I was asked to address the members and set out my ideas as to what we should be seeking to achieve and any thoughts I might have regarding the strategies and tactics we should adopt in order to achieve them provided, of course, that everyone present was in agreement with my suggestions. These were basically that we should do all in our power to build maximum public participation in the manner in which services were run and administered and, where possible and practicable, to devolve the administration of the services to the user groups with a light handed overview from members and officers. In addition we should seek to increase the range and provision of services year on year to the maximum allowed under the financial resources available.

This found favour and the suggestion that I should stand for Leader was advanced. I pointed out that this was not practical since I needed to learn the ways of Local Government as all my experience hitherto was in the Trade Union movement although I did have some experience of Chairmanship. I also pointed out that the recent group meeting had, I believed, demonstrated a noticeable shortcoming in that area.

Thus it came about that some three months later, following two Council meetings at which I successfully challenged the Mayor's (Council Chair) decisions on procedure, together with two lengthy group meetings, I found myself elected as Chair of the Labour group.

On a day-to-day basis, when any issue arose which was outside the range of any decisions already endorsed by a vote at a full Council meeting, the Council was run by the General Purposes Sub-Committee of the Policy and Resources Committee. This sub-committee consisted of four members, the Chair and Vice Chair of the Policy and Resources Committee who in turn were also Leader and Deputy Leader of the Council, and their equivalents from the largest minority party. This struck me as incongruous and an effective block on decision making since with an even number of members from opposite sides of the fence, there existed the potential for permanent stalemate when it came to decision making. I therefore approached the Borough Solicitor to establish if this situation was a matter of Local Government law or simply a local custom, arguing that the committee should be made up of an odd number in order to be really effective. He assured me that the composition of the General Purposes Sub-Committee was not laid down in Local Government law and that there was validity in my argument. Provided such a change was endorsed by a full Council decision it was perfectly valid.

So, after gaining the support of the Labour group, I put forward a motion that would increase the General Purposes Sub-Committee to five members, the fifth of whom would be the Chair of the majority group. Somewhat to my surprise, following a unanimous vote, some thirteen months later after my election onto the Council, I found myself, effectively if not openly, in control politically of the organisation.

After the second A.G.M. of my Council tenure I became a member of the Policy and Resources Committee, dropping membership of Housing. It was at this point, I believe, that the Directors and Chief Officers began to become wary of me and I was frequently quoted and referred to in media reports of Council meetings. On numerous occasions I had placed the Tories in embarrassing situations when I would amend the motions they placed before Council with minor adjustments to the wording which would completely changed their original intention and objectives. These amendments were then carried on a Labour vote so further securing their embarrassment by forcing them to vote against their own resolutions.

This embarrassment however was not always one way. The Tory Leader, in the early 1980s, was somewhat sharper than most of his colleagues. At a full Council meeting one evening, following a question directed at the then Leader who was inclined to give long rambling and not too clever responses, having received no precise answer the Tory Leader enquired if perhaps the Deputy Leader could assist. The Leader declined to respond so the Tory Leader, still smarting from the changed situation with the General Purposes Sub-Committee, then asked the Mayor, who that year had been a Tory nominee, if he would ask the "real Leader" of the Council to answer. The Mayor initially hesitated then, glancing at the Tory Leader, caught his drift and looked around the room at the forty nine Councillors present, firmly fixing his gaze at the top corner where I was sitting and asked me if I would give the explanation that the Councillors were seeking.

In the two years between 1980 and 1983 a number of wards which had previously had an allocation of two Local Authority seats acquired a third seat which had the effect of strengthening the hand of the Trotskyite element on the Swindon G.M.C. since they controlled the nomination of Councillors. As a result, whilst group meetings were now usually concluded by 10.30 p.m., they were more contentious. This was because, taking advantage of the right of the Chair to sum up discussions and explain the two sides in any contentious discussions I could always, with the added advantage of the casting vote, ensure their attempts to dictate policy were defeated which annoyed them intensely. The old guard, eventually coming to realise that their day had passed, would invariably follow my lead in voting, regarding that as the lesser of two evils, but the Stratton element adamantly clung to what power they still had,

In 1983 the current Leader who, many years earlier himself occupied the position of young pretender, decided to accept nomination to the Mayorship therefore relinquishing his leadership role.

Throughout this period, other than the occasional need to eat a snack, usually a KitKat or similar, during a meeting, the diabetes caused little problem. I had wisely ensured that my colleagues and most of those officers I was involved with knew of my diabetic condition.

With the date of the A.G.M. approaching my A.E.U. colleague had contacted most group members sounding them out with regard to supporting my nomination for the leadership. This was something I was then, nor ever have been, prepared to do myself. It was obviously going to prove difficult since I was anathema to the Trotskyite section, more so since I continuously frustrated their best laid plans having, in my industrial experience, seen them all before. So it came to pass that in order to secure power the leadership went to an elderly Councillor even more sedate and rambling in Council meetings than the former occupant. I attained the post of Deputy Leader and became, in effect, the "power behind the throne".

The officers and the media quickly became aware of the reality and whilst paying due respect and courtesy to the holder of the office, invariably directed any enquiries for guidance on policy or requests for interviews or comment at me. In 1983, when Thamesdown became one of the seventeen Local Authorities to be rate capped, these media requests became increasingly frequent.

As a consequence of being Deputy Leader I automatically became Chair of the Development Sub-Committee whose remit covered the acquisition and control of all the Council's land assets, rents on commercial assets and their acquisition or disposal. I was also Vice Chair of the Policy and Resources Committee.

In addition to these posts I also chaired the Direct Labour Sub-Committee and setting out to expand the scope and efficiency of our Direct Labour Organisation was an early objective. With the employment of a Manager from the building industry, together with my own background in that industry, this objective was soon achieved. Having set up a double glazing production unit we were soon in a position of beating the private sector in competitive tenders for the provision of double glazing and electrical services across a host of other Local Authorities, much to the chagrin of the local Tory M.P. and ultimately Maggie Thatcher's government who in 1983 placed Thamesdown on the hit list of rate capped Local Authorities.

Thamesdown was one of only two District Councils, the other being Basildon in Essex, which had been built post 1945 as a new town with all its construction and development costs borne by the Government. Swindon, or Thamesdown as the borough rather than the town was known then, had however received none of that Central Government help. Post 1945 the far sighted Local Authority, blessed with an astute Town Clerk and a Council Leader of similar acumen, had become concerned that Swindon was in essence, at that time, a one industry town based on Brunel's G.W.R. works and, as an expanding town had taken on the role of a growth area.

With the desperate housing situation pertaining in London due to the loss of housing stock between 1939 and 1945, Thamesdown struck a deal with the then London County Council which initiated the town's expansion. This involved a partial release of funding, but by no means all, which saw the town's area and population grow by a third between 1945 and 1960.

All the other threatened Councils under the legislation proposed were Metropolitan Authorities, i.e. big cities or districts. The legislation was due to take effect in 1984 and in the latter part of 1983 those Authorities targeted on the Government's hit list, came together in London to discuss tactics and strategy. There were initially twenty Local Authorities on this hit list out of which five eventually decided to comply.

At that first meeting it was hugely apparent that Thamesdown's Leader, who had sat mute and somewhat perplexed throughout, was clearly out of his depth, leaving it to me, his Deputy, to explain our situation and position. It was also clear that he was not alone in this regard and at all subsequent meetings both Thamesdown and Liverpool were represented by their respective Deputy Leaders.

Meanwhile, at local level, we had, in Thamesdown, a Chief Officer whose remit it was to seek and attract companies to the town who would supply much needed employment. Prior to his employment in Local Government, this man had been employed by the City of London and, by inclination, was a "dyed in the wool" capitalist. The tenure of his reports to the Development Sub-Committee, of which I was Chair, were, to me, like a red rag to a bull. He was constantly putting forward recommendations to reduce rental and lease-hold charges to retail and commercial leases of Council property. He was also frequently seeking freehold disposal of Council land assets. I had to forcefully point out to him, on a number of occasions, that our aim was to maximise receipts from the private sector for the benefit of the people of the town and that we had little faith in the concept that future wealth depended on the so-called service economy. This was very much a misconception which, in the current situation now in 2010, has been thoroughly justified and proven my analysis at that time to have been correct. Much to the relief of a number of the officers he realised he had no chance of convincing me, a devout socialist, that there was any merit to his reports.

However it wasn't until he made another attempt at submitting a ridiculous proposal that he finally realised his often self declared talents were not appreciated and followed my advice that he should perhaps take them elsewhere and quit. This was when he tried to get permission for a private air taxi service to operate from a strip close to what had once been the Vickers aircraft factory on the eastern periphery of the town. He had rather stupidly gone public with his proposal prior to presenting a report to committee and when he did present his report it was thoroughly trashed and thrown out.

There was yet another problem on the horizon at this time when, as Thatcher's policies increasingly began to bite and with unemployment mounting, the influence of the Trotskyites began to assert itself. This took the usual form of impossible demands and a concentration on attacking Labour administrations, irrespective of whether their stance was left, they would never be left enough for the Trotskyites, or right which strangely drew less criticism!

In London in the 1950s the epithet "Hampstead Socialists" was coined. These individuals usually adopted a patronising and somewhat paternalistic attitude assuming, wrongly, that the workers were not capable of organising or vocalising grievances and were therefore in constant need of their guidance and assistance. My own perception and experience of working class history and struggle however was the complete opposite of this. The vast majority of working class people were only too aware of the daily struggle necessary to feed and house their families and had little time for these alleged sympathisers who had no conception of the complexities of their struggles. What is more the working class had very little regard for those not prepared to pull their weight and those who just could not be bothered. Anyone reading this who has worked in a factory or establishment wherever large numbers of people are performing the same or similar tasks will know of such individuals.

In 1983 things came to a head in Swindon when there emerged a body called "The Swindon Unemployed Movement". Their main spokesman was a man who was unknown to anyone in the Labour movement until the sudden appearance of leaflets from this group. Additionally, around this time, I was made aware of a meeting that was due to take place one evening in Gloucester, news of which was leaked to me by one of the officers. This meeting was to be addressed by the Rail Workshops National Personnel Director. I therefore persuaded the Council Leader that he should plead a prior engagement so that I, as Deputy Leader, could attend in his stead.

The meeting took place in Tudor style manor houses outside Gloucester and attendees consisted of members from Regional Employers Associations, Chambers of Commerce, and representatives/officers from Local Government. Our arrival caused the B.R.E.L. Personnel Director some concern on the basis that the information he would be imparting must, by its very nature, be regarded as private and confidential. He felt that in view of the fact that I was a B.R.E.L. employee this could well restrict the amount of information he would be able to impart. However a fellow Councillor from Gloucestershire County Council made it clear to him that I, as Deputy Leader of a Council as large and regionally significant as Thamesdown, would be familiar with the concept of private and confidential but I also had a duty of responsibility to its citizens. Therefore he should proceed with the meeting's agenda as planned which he reluctantly did.

From his statement it soon became clear to me that there were two immediate implications for Swindon. First was the closure of the apprentice training school and secondly the proposed 1,200 redundancies as a consequence of the reorganisation and contraction of the rail works. However of prime importance was the potential closure of the works within the next five years.

These last two announcements came as no surprise to me since I had been part of the team originally involved in the reorganisation of the works and was well able to anticipate the political and economic moves being adopted by the Tory Government. It struck me there were two things we, as a Local Authority, could do. Firstly we needed to take responsibility, on an arm's length basis, and take over the Rail Apprentice Training School should it become available and secondly to increase the Council's own apprentice intake. Both these proposals achieved unanimous support when placed before a meeting of the full Council and yet were condemned by the Swindon Unemployed Movement as being contrary to their interests.

Another odd situation emerged when many men in the works became increasingly concerned at the lack of information emanating from the Works Committee. They were constantly questioning me on what the Council knew with regard to the future of the works or the land which it occupied. There was additionally some concern expressed by many about what appeared to them to be a close relationship between certain members of the Works Committee and the B.R.E.L. Personnel Director. So, in order to explain the Council's position, I drafted an open letter to the Works Committee and shop floor workers with a request that it be clearly displayed on all shop notice boards. The following day this resulted in the ridiculous situation that after my letter had been posted onto notice boards by members of the Works Committee those members whose perceived relationship had been the cause of concern were then going round and taking them down.

In the meantime the Trotskyite element amongst the Councillors was seeking to set up a Working Party to assist any campaign that may emerge in resistance of possible redundancies within the rail works. This was a perfect example of the patronizing paternalism that I have referred to earlier. Here were a group of professional Social Workers and their acolytes thinking themselves able to lead or assist the historically most experienced and advanced group of workers in the locality whose forebears had created the whole social and intellectual foundation of the town since the mid 1800s. The arrogance of this assumption took my breath away.

Some eighteen months previously this group had been extremely disconcerted when I turned up at a public meeting they had organised. There were numerous murmurs of disapproval as I entered the room and began to walk down the aisle to find a seat. This mood soon turned to stunned amazement when the main speaker, who was about to be introduced, caught sight of me and promptly leapt off the platform and advanced up the aisle to meet me where we immediately threw our arms around each other in a fraternal hug. This was no other than Gerry Gable, now editor of the anti-facist magazine, "Searchlight" who, twenty years earlier in London, had been my good friend when we worked as a contracting pair.

Knowing I had moved to Swindon in 1961, which had been the reason we had ceased to work as a pair, when he had received the invitation to attend this meeting, Gerry had asked one of his researchers to endeavour to make contact with me after he had been informed that I was heavily involved with the local Council. Gerry had subsequently contacted my P.A. to advise her he would be attending. I had no prior knowledge that the meeting was even taking place since, I believe, that efforts had been made to keep me in ignorance of it.

The meeting organisers were not at all pleased to find their star speaker was so close to their main Labour group opponent even though the main purpose of the meeting was to create an anti-racism alliance which I wholeheartedly approved of!

During this period, sometime in 1982, when walking around the town with Joan, I had occasion to visit the Director of Arts & Recreation and I asked her if she would accompany me as I anticipated my visit would not take long after which we could resume our agenda. Joan agreed to this as it would give her the opportunity for a welcome cup of tea. With business concluded the Director turned to Joan and expressed his wish that she would allow me to continue as a Councillor. He emphasised that both he and his colleagues acknowledged that in me they received a clear and consistent lead and guidance and whilst it was taking some adjusting to was nevertheless much appreciated. He for one was convinced I would one day aspire to Leader of the Council. Joan responded that provided the stress involved did not have any adverse effects on my diabetes then she would raise no objections or stand in my way.

A clear boost for Labour

4.5.84

LABOUR leaders in Thamesdown will be delighted at the results of yesterday's council election — even though the narrow margin by which deputy leader Tony Huzzey won his seat must have given them a nasty scare.

The party has gained one seat overall in Thamesdown council. And it is clear from the general pattern of voting that the council's policy of continued expansion, and of strongly fighting the Government's rate-capping and other proposals, has not lost Labour any support. Far from it.

The dreadful news of the impending closure of the British Rail Engineering Works must have damaged Conservative interests, for it is an inevitable conclusion that the run-down of the works is a direct result of the Government's refusal to invest properly in British Rail, even though it may be that for internal political reasons the Swindon works is being picked off while other BREL centres are being treated more favourably.

Losing ground

On the national front, as Mrs Thatcher celebrates five years as Prime Minister, she has certainly not got the anniversary presents from the voters she was looking for. The only thing that might cheer her is that two more women MPs — one Conservative and one Labour — will now join the scandalously small number in the commons.

All three parties can take some comfort from the local election results but the general picture is bad for the Government. The Conservatives were bound to lose some ground since they were defending seats won in the swing to them after the Falklands War. Nevertheless, Labour will be pleased to have won such major cities as Birmingham and Edinburgh.

The challenge to the government squeeze on local government spending will become stronger. Labour will argue that the voters have strengthened the case against Mr Jenkin's plans for rate-capping.

The clear message of these election results to Mrs Thatcher is that the country does not want drastic cuts in public services or a Conservative party that swings still further to the right.

Indication of support of Thamesdown electorate for anti rate-cap stance.

Political and Health Stress Combated

As the stress increased, particularly during the next two years, what with combating the threat of rate capping and the constant struggle of inhibiting the attempts of the Trotskyite group to undermine the fight back against the Government's manoeuvres, the one person I could always rely upon without exception was my wonderful wife, coupled with a great home life. She never complained, despite the fact that my evenings, from May 1980 to 1990, were always spent on Council business with the exception perhaps once a quarter when I would re-arrange meetings to allow me to accompany her to a skittles match. She and her colleagues were part of a team in the Civil Service League and we enjoyed those occasional evenings out. We were equally happy to be alone in our own company and it was her constant love and support and the secure home environment she provided that kept me focused and intent on my role and objectives.

The early discussions of those rate capped Authorities centred on determining what common objectives we shared, the means of achieving them and the tactics and strategies to be employed. One of the first decisions taken was the appointment of a spokesperson who would also be Chair and we elected David Blunkett, the blind Sheffield Leader, to this position. We sought common ground on a number of points to place, initially, before Patrick Jenkins, the then Environment Secretary. This brought to light some basic differences of approach which were subsequently enhanced by Liverpool, the main dissenting Authority, which like Thamesdown was represented in the main by its Deputy Leader, a man named Derek Hatton. He later achieved some notoriety over the course of the next few months following a meeting with Patrick Jenkins which achieved nothing other than to confirm our suspicions that come hell or high water the Government was intent on implementing the legislation which would effectively remove the right of Local Authorities to set a budget that would allow them to follow the policies on which they were elected.

This would obviously have a devastating effect, so far as Thamesdown was concerned. In the financial year 1983-1984 the Local Authority budget was £15 million but the Tory Government set the target for the financial year 1984-1985 at £13.6 million taking no account of inflation. This amounted to an 86% reduction in spending but we were determined there would be no cuts in jobs or services.

So the course was set for a confrontation which was to last for the next five years. In fact Thamesdown became the only Council to be rate capped from beginning to end of that legislation. We had, however, three things in our favour. Although I say it myself, these were a determined and reasonably adroit political leadership, a highly skilled and committed Borough Treasurer and the support of the local electorate and media.

In the first year we undertook a campaign to inform the public of the borough about the full implications of the legislation and its impact on the quality of life they enjoyed insofar as their cultural and recreational facilities were concerned and the potential threat to environmental health and surroundings. For example Thamesdown had extensive grass verges running alongside the main dual carriageways that bisected the town's expanding estates. These had historically been cut regularly each Spring but now turned from green to yellow. The cut back on grass cutting also totally hid the legend "Spring has sprung" which was spelt out by strategically planted daffodils on the grass mound at junction 16 off the M4. This had achieved international interest and attention and was much appreciated by the populace.

The murals that were painted by a local artist on gable end houses across the town, ably assisted by volunteers from amongst the local youth group, together with the dance and media studios and workshop, gave many of the town's unemployed youngsters opportunities to develop their skills. Many of these initiatives had come about over the four years following my election onto the Council in 1980.

I had expressed an interest in the Arts & Recreation Committee and at the first committee meeting I attended a paper had been presented expressing the objective of opening up the arts to public participation. The Director of that committee was recommending its rejection. This paper had attracted my attention because it encapsulated all my own thoughts on providing opportunities to individuals to realise their full potential. I perceived that the author of this paper was probably from the same background and also held similar beliefs to myself. I managed to convince the committee to initially reject the Director's recommendation and to allow the author to address the committee. The Director was reluctant to agree to this but his body language caused me to cast my eyes over the group of junior officers assembled around the periphery of the room one of whom, obviously the said author, was clearly indicating his reluctance to speak. I therefore switched to a different tactic and asked that the report be deferred to a subsequent meeting and with mutual agreement the meeting then closed.

As the mass of officers and members left the room I managed to waylay the reluctant officer. He, however, maintains that I actually pinned him against the wall in the corridor. A big man, in a denim jacket, he was about five feet eight inches tall to my six feet one inch and my recollection of that incident is somewhat different. I can remember him shyly endeavouring to edge aside a curtain in order to dodge the Director's line of sight in the Committee Room. However on one aspect of that night we are both agreed. Terry Court, the officer concerned, and I were both from an ordinary working class background and, prior to attending college and taking an Arts Degree, he had briefly been an apprentice electrician and was a convinced socialist. Over the course of the next decade both he and I expanded the initiative he had originally started as a young junior school Arts Teacher which was a project whereby the children at Christmas either made gifts or took part in fund raising for local pensioners. This, together with Terry's management skills and my subsequent political support, had evolved into a body called Thamesdown Community Arts which encapsulated all our ideas. This group was democratically run by its members with professional support and guidance available if required and requested. Funding was provided by both the public sector, i.e. Southern Arts and Thamesdown Borough Council and also the private sector, i.e. Hambro Life and Burmah Castrol.

The Thamesdown Community Arts Studio gave rise to a host of entrants to the Ballet Rambert and Sadlers Wells including a number of renowned choreographers and also the Media Lab who subsequently established careers in the television and film industry. Indeed either the Producer or the Director of the Harry Potter trilogy was a former pupil of the Thamesdown Community Arts Media Lab.

On one occasion a touch of California was brought to Swindon when one night at the local speedway stadium car park we set up a drive-in cinema. An early technical hitch initially caused us some concern but this was soon overcome and the experience was a great success. Even Joan, whose first thought was that perhaps I had had a hypo when I supported and indeed pushed the enterprise through, admitted it had been a very enjoyable experience and acknowledged it had been a tremendous success.

On another occasion Hambro Life, whose Managing Director was Joel Joffe, later to become Lord Joffe, who was himself an ardent and committed supporter, had asked that we organise the Swindon Hambro Festival the cost of which the company would cover. This was to take place in a marquee in a park in the centre of the town and was organised entirely by the Council. The event was to feature both classical and popular music, dance and drama and international acts amongst whom where the Count Basie Band, the London Symphony Orchestra and the Moscow State Circus.

Unfortunately for me I was in hospital at the time awaiting an operation following a stroke. At my suggestion an approach had been made to Ella Fitzgerald and I can remember receiving a call from Terry Court telling me that unfortunately she had to cancel her appearance due to illness. She had been due to appear with Count Basie and the show was obviously completely sold out so he asked me if I could suggest an alternative. I advised him that he might like to try Cleo Laine who subsequently accepted and duly appeared in place of Ella Fitzgerald. Confined to hospital in Oxford as I was, I sadly missed that performance. However I consoled myself with the thought that in either 1954 or 1955 I had been in attendance at the Royal Festival Hall at what I believe was Cleo Laine's first public appearance with the Dankworth Seven. I had received a ticket for this performance addressed to myself at home in Peckham which, to this day, now sixty years later, I still do not know from whom. I had gone to the performance on the night fully expecting to see someone I knew seated nearby but that was not the case and it was then and still is a mystery but one that was very much appreciated.

Whilst still adhering to our socialist principles, the Labour Council's successful relationship with the private sector did nothing other than cause the Tories, both locally and nationally, extreme aggravation, but the electorate thought it was great.

It was whilst attending the launch of one of these public and private sector initiatives, albeit a minor one, that I was approached by the wife of one of my councillor colleagues who told me that her husband harboured ambitions to take my job as Leader. I responded that his chance would come as I would not be seeking re-election to the Council two years hence.

I was later approached by the councillor himself who told me that he thought we had much in common. Puzzled at this remark I pointed out to him that he came from an affluent middle class background, had attended university and was now an academic working in research for a government financed international body whereas I came from a working class family, had served an apprenticeship and worked as a skilled tradesman so I queried what had led him to come that conclusion. He responded that we had both been Y.C. members in our youth. I asked him if he had not missed off a letter and received a negative response. At this I pointed out that I had been a member of the Young Communist League not the Young Conservatives! Somewhat taken aback at that he withdrew knowing that he had now revealed to me his past affiliations. He did however eventually achieve his ambition.

To return to the situation following the implementation of the rate capping legislation, Liverpool received little support from amongst the group of Local Authorities so targeted. This consisted, in the main, of the three South London Boroughs. It was with some surprise to them that the person advancing alternative strategies, i.e. myself, but with the same objectives of resistance, spoke in the same accent as themselves but represented, in their view, an obscure little Authority in the South West. However outside of Committee I assured them that I did indeed I originate from their own neck of the woods which overcame their possible suspicions towards me and the line I was pushing in opposition to the Liverpool one was accepted.

In the Thamesdown Labour Group, whilst they were not members of the militant sector, there was a small group of about three people who voiced some sympathy with the militant line. So, at the 1984 A.G.M., I contested the leadership but not being successful declined to stand for the position of Deputy which ultimately went to one of those three. The Labour Group however insisted that I continue to represent Thamesdown in the rate capped Local Authority discussions when the newly elected Deputy expressed a reluctance to do so. I believe he was a Partner in a local Employment and Recruitment Agency and whether or not that influenced his decision to resign the position some six months later or not I cannot say.

Again I stood aside and another of the three was elected to the position. Unfortunately he, like myself, also had a chronic illness which I believe perhaps inhibited his performance to a greater degree than my own.

In the 1985 group election however, having again by a tactical alignment of the right and so-called militant left element, I lost out once more to the former and older established man who had, two years earlier, by a similar left and right cohesion, been elected as Leader. These elections were always very close and there were never more than four votes between us. However, after the self proclaimed left for one reason or another had not been able to cover the Deputy position adequately, I again stood and was finally elected with a clear, across the board, result even in the face of opposition from Tory, Liberal and Social Democrat officers.

My election to this position was also much to the relief of the woman who acted as P.A. to the Chief Executive, Leader and Deputy, who, in much consternation and some embarrassment, had to explain to the previous Leader that his name was constantly being rejected by the media, i.e. newspapers, radio and T.V., who always specified my name over his in their approaches for interviews/statements.

It also caused me some embarrassment at work where, in my post of Chief Electrical Maintenance Foreman, I had to carry a bleeper so that I could be easily contacted in cases of any breakdown. When it went off through the mid 1980s, I would contact the works telephone switchboard to establish the location of the problem and the girls answering my call would respond that all was O.K. and it was merely a request for the media star. They assured me that no sarcasm was intended but I am sure they enjoyed their little joke. To the constant irritation of Joan and my mother I would appear in front of the T.V. cameras dressed in either a T-shirt or donkey jacket, depending upon the prevailing weather conditions at the time.

On the political front in 1983 or 1984, Neil Kinnock, the then Leader of the Opposition, came to Swindon on a political tour and, together with the Council Leader, I joined them on a tour round the town which ultimately ended with a visit to the rail works. The Leader had never actually worked in the rail works which was quite unusual for a man of his age, i.e. 70+, and trade, in a town that was dominated by such a big employer during his working life. So it was left to me to accompany Neil Kinnock to and around the works.

The journey from our location in the north of the town through to the works at Rodbourne was quite a unique experience, it being decided I should accompany him in his car which I believe was driven by an officer from the Special Branch. We were preceded by a police patrol car with sirens blaring and lights flashing through crowded thoroughfares crammed with traffic which was forced aside as we shot through at speed. I was stupefied, thinking if this was how the citizenry were pushed aside for the Leader of the Opposition then how much worse would it be for the public had it been the Prime Minister – complete road closure?

The visit itself went well and I was able to answer to Neil Kinnock's satisfaction the numerous questions, observations and queries that he put to me. At the end of the visit, having covered a considerable number of subjects in our discussions, he asked me if I had considered putting myself forward for selection as prospective M.P. to which I categorically replied that I had not. He responded that I should do so as he felt there was a great need in Parliament for politically aware and skilled genuine working class people like myself who had been educated by my own experience of working life and Local Government which was increasingly dominated by graduates with very little life experience. If I succeeded in getting onto the list of candidates then he would ensure I got a winnable seat. I responded that I felt I could achieve more for the people of Thamesdown in my current position than would be possible in Parliament which already subjected me to a great deal of stress with the constant reports and papers I had to read, not to mention the endless meetings, media interviews and the additional stress of keeping the group together.

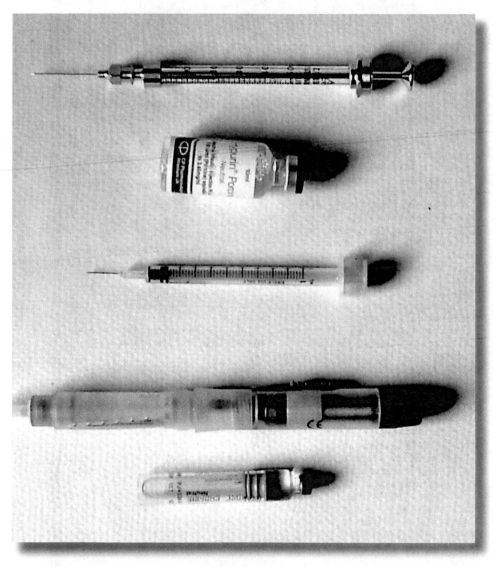

Syringes and Insulin vials – is this all that 50 years research has achieved?

29-11-88

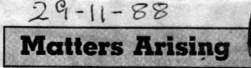

Matters Arising

NEIL MERRICK takes a light-hearted look at local government.

Who'll be front runner for '89?

Who will be leader of Thamesdown Council next year? Tony Huzzey? Ricky Midwinter? Or how about Simon Cordon?

Coun Cordon has emerged from the obscurity of a little party called the SDP to become favourite to lead Thamesdown's controlling Labour group.

This follows his amazing achievement at last week's meeting of the policy and resources committee.

Councillors were discussing next year's budget and — as usual — Coun Huzzey was getting an unfair share of hassle from Labour's so-called West Swindon Tendency.

Consisting of Coun Midwinter and community planning chairman Tony Free, the West Swindon Tendency has a carefully thought out policy — it disagrees with Coun Huzzey on everything.

The two rascals dared to abstain when Coun Huzzey's much-heralded City deal was being discussed a few weeks ago, even though the deal appears to have solved Thamesdown's immediate cash crisis.

Last week, they continued to press the Labour leader over his plans for the future disposal of land assets.

What was the matter with them? Were they just jealous about not being invited to London to meet John Selwyn Gummer or had they forgotten this was not a behind-closed-doors Labour group meeting?

In the face of such open defiance, Coun Huzzey just smiled and pressed ahead with the business to hand. He looked more self-assured after having put on a suit for the first time in his life.

Membership of the West Swindon Tendency is expanding since public works chairman Derique Montaut waved goodbye to Moredon and moved into his new house in Shaw.

But few people trust Coun Montaut's motives for asking Coun Huzzey about plans to sell more land in West Swindon.

They think he is simply afraid the council will try to flog his back garden.

But where does Coun Cordon come into all this, you are probably thinking?

Well, the SDP councillor apologised for spoiling the occasion but, he said, he was forced to point out there seemed to be some disagreement within the Labour group.

That was it. Labour councillors needed no further encouragement.

They were not going to put up with Coun Cordon accusing them of being divided.

Within a few seconds, Coun Cordon managed to achieve something neither Coun Huzzey nor Coun Midwinter have managed in the past five years.

He had united the Labour group!

Speculation on internal divisions in the Labour group

Left wingers lashed in power struggle

9.5.84

By JUSTIN DAVENPORT

A FIERCE political row broke out today over the leadership election of Thamesdown Council.

Left-wingers on the Labour-controlled borough were accused of siding with the right to achieve their own ends, leaving the moderates out in the cold.

And Coun. Tony Huzzey attacked the Left for putting personal ambition before the interests of local people.

The storm erupted after a shock decision to vote veteran moderate councillor Arthur Miles back into power as leader last night.

He pulled off a surprise win over his deputy Coun. Huzzey during a secret ballot for the position within Thamesdown's Labour group.

Coun. Huzzey, who regained his Covingham seat by just nine votes in last week's council elections, was strongly tipped to take over the position.

But he was narrowly defeated after Coun. Miles was proposed for the leadership by Left-winger Coun. Malcolm Sargeant.

Coun. Huzzey himself was also only re-elected as deputy after a contest for the position with Coun. Sargeant.

And afterwards he accused the left of engineering the result.

"They have amalgamated with the right in a bid to gain power. They are aiming to break through to gain control as a result of this," declared Coun. Huzzey.

He claimed that Labour's policies to improve life for people in Swindon would now be put in jeopardy.

But Labour's internal group chairman Coun. Jim D'Aila denied there was any split within the party.

There were few other surprises in the contests which decide the membership and chairmanship of committees.

Controversial councillor Les Gowing, who recently proposed that a council brothel should be set up in Swindon, was ousted from his position as housing chairman.

Tied

Coun. Derek Montaut, who also made the news recently by buying his own council home, was elected in his place — on the toss of a coin.

He and Coun. D'Avila twice tied for the position of housing chairman.

And the only member qualified to put a casting vote was Coun. D'Avila himself — as the newly-elected leader of the internal group.

Said Coun. D'Avila afterwards: "It was highly embarrassing that it was so close. I did not want to use my casting vote so we decided on the toss of a coin.

"This has never happened before within the group, but it was quite amicable."

Coun. Eammon Hackett takes charge of the arts and recreation committee following the decision by the previous chairman Tony Mayer to step down as a councillor.

But there was no change at the top of the community planning committees where councillors Ricky Midwinter and Peter Gallagher stay on as chairmen.

Failure to capture Thamesdown Council leadership

••• 189 •••

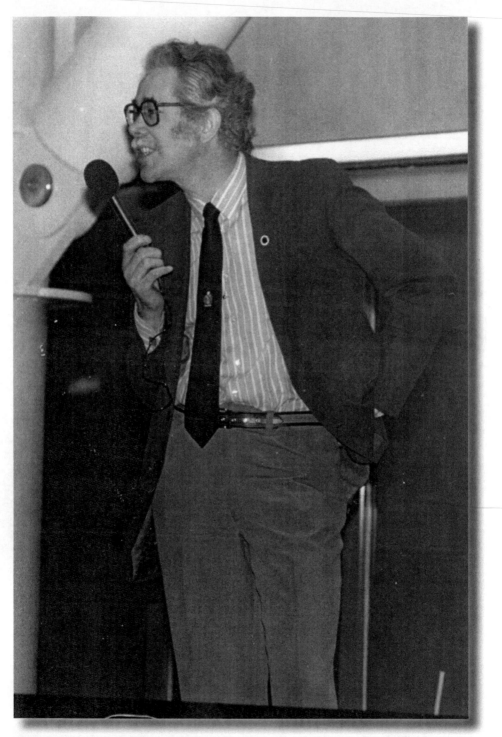

Addressing the crowd at the opening of the Swindon Link Centre, built
at no cost to rate payers by Council financial arrangements 26 April 1985

Insulin Changes and Honda Acquisition

The medical profession now bought forward, under the influence of the drug industry, radical changes in the provision of insulin. Until 1984 insulin had been available in three strengths, i.e. twenty, forty and eighty units per cc. It was claimed that too many mistakes were being made by patients in the administration of their insulin. This was nonsense. Having been dependant on the degree of their requirement for insulin, patients were always subscribed the required amount at the appropriate strength and providing they had originally been correctly assessed with regard to their requirement then that was the amount they would have injected each and everyday of their lives. Unless their respective GPs had made a mistake in their prescription they would not administer the incorrect strength.

The other possible area of potential error in the administration of insulin was if the diabetic concerned was hospitalised, in which case their dosage would probably be administered by someone other than themselves, i.e. a nurse or a doctor. Therefore any problems with administration of insulin were more likely to be the responsibility of the medical profession and not the patient.

However the decision was taken to standardise the strength of insulin at one hundred units per cc. This, we were told, was as a result of international agreement, yet another example of deliberate misinformation as neither Germany nor France put it into operation until many years later.

In the case of those of us who were, in particular, on bovine eighty units per cc insulin, this caused tremendous problems and from one end of the country to the other both the local and national press carried alarming and tragic stories of the problems that arose as a result of this change.

There was also a second element of **deliberate false information** that was then circulated, initially to the medical profession. This was that due to the spreading vegetarianism amongst citizens of the developed countries and the resultant decrease in beef and pork consumption, animal insulins would no longer be available so therefore a human insulin would be introduced. This had been genetically engineered using yeast and bacteria and was claimed to be an exact reproduction of the insulin produced by non-diabetics.

These developments were not introduced in any way whatsoever for the benefit of the diabetic but were solely for the benefit of the drug companies whose unit costs in insulin production were reduced and whose profit per prescription soared, as I was subsequently to prove, after persistent requests and questions to the Ministry of Health who, for some time, refused to respond.

The standardisation of insulin strength brought about, for me, the most disconcerting period in the management and control of my diabetes that I had ever experienced in the nearly forty years since my diagnosis. What is more, it enhanced Joan's concerns and for that fact alone I will never forgive or trust the drug companies again. Despite their protestations to the contrary all they were and are primarily concerned with is profit, not the provision of better health care.

Despite this further pressure on my ability to perform my role as Deputy Leader, I carried out the task but, as was now clearly obvious to everyone, the current Leader was just not up to the job. This was now a critical stage for the Council as we were confronted with a Government restriction on expenditure of £13.6 million even though our pre-capped budget had been £15 million which had been set the previous year. We were faced with real problems just to maintain our existing level of services let alone expand them and uphold our promise to the electorate in this regard. Absolutely no account had been taken of the ensuing inflation of the past twelve months.

Prior to setting the budget, the Chief Executive of the Council asked me if I would accompany the Leader and himself to the A.G.M. of the Association of District Councils in Bournemouth. There was a matter he wished to discuss which directly involved myself as Chair of the Development Sub-Committee. I was intrigued that he had felt it necessary to remove ourselves from Swindon in order to discuss this and after checking with Joan that she would be OK if I went away for a couple of nights, upon which she remarked with a grin that she would feel cold but would appreciate the rest and an undisturbed couple of nights' sleep, I agreed to go.

Our stay on that first night, with dinner and a couple of bottles of Mosel wine between the three of us, was an experience which really brought home to me the difference between the classes in the U.K. My proportion of the cost for just that one meal probably came very close to a week's wages of a skilled man. Yet there were people who dined like that every night and I still, to this day, cannot see how that could possibly be justified.

The next day, over a lunch of dressed crab, I was told that a major Japanese company had approached the Council in order to assess the response they were likely to receive if they chose Swindon to develop a manufacturing facility from the four locations in the country they were considering. From our questioning of the Chief Executive, it emerged that the company wanted to install a pre-delivery inspection facility with the long term possibility of an engine production facility and, if all went well regarding the U.K. relationship with the European Union, ultimately a full vehicle assembly plant. However, under no circumstances whatsoever could this information be revealed because if it became public knowledge then they would withdraw.

We established the identity of the company in question and knowing full well that the closure of the town's rail works was now imminent, I immediately gave my agreement for the Council to issue a positive response to the Japanese. However I had a nasty shock a week later when, after a meeting of the Development Sub-Committee, I was apprehended by the Local Government reporter from the local newspaper who insisted we go for a drink.

Contrary to the belief that reporters can drink their source of information under the table in order to get their story, I succeeded in reversing the situation. The reporter was less than half my age and seemed to know of a potential big development in the town. I was desperate to establish just how much he knew and from where his information had come from. He knew nothing of any consequences of such a story being made public but what he did know he had apparently been told by the Leader of the Tory group. This man had a habit, when the occasion arose, of going into the Chief Executive's office on some pretext or other in an attempt to read any correspondence on his desk or diary entries but in substance he was just fishing for information.

The following morning I contacted the Editor and cautioned him that any speculation appearing in the papers could have dire consequences and I promised him a national exclusive if and when we had anything to reveal. However any printed speculation would guarantee there would be nothing. The Editor asked what I was going to do about the person who had given this information to his reporter whom, he cynically stated, had been foolish enough to reveal his information source to me. I assured him that I would deal with it having established that nothing material to this potential acquisition would be committed to paper.

So I duly confronted the Tory Leader and told him I now definitely knew the source of the occasional leak of private and confidential information to the press and I would have no hesitation in revealing it. He bridled at this and said he knew of my previous political affiliation to which I responded that I had never hidden this information and indeed it was common knowledge.

However, with regard to Honda, having secured the necessary secrecy surrounding their initial approach, we successfully completed discussions with them which, in the course of succeeding years, eventually gave rise to the establishment of the manufacturing plant that exists in Swindon today. This proved to be, I believe, the last truly significant employment enhancing company to relocate to the town.

About a year or so earlier I had devised and drawn up a resolution on the subject of Council house sales which sought to recognise the intentions of the Tory Government in that regard. This "right to buy" had certainly caused a large number of previous Labour voters to switch their allegiance to the Tories. Rather than just putting up blind opposition my resolution would give Local Authorities the right to build houses for sale or rent in order to meet demand in their area and so hopefully negate the need to sell off Council housing stock. This was to be achieved using Central Government finance advanced to the Local Authorities at an agreed rate of interest that was fixed at 0.5% - 1.5% above the Bank rate at the time of the loan. Furthermore, Local Authorities should also be given control of all development land in their area.

This was adopted by the Devizes constituency G.M.C. and I was appointed their delegate to that year's Labour Party Conference in Blackpool. On the Saturday afternoon, prior to the start of the conference the following Monday, together with a host of other delegates I was brought before the Conference Arrangements Committee with the view to amalgamating resolutions on similar subject matters into composites to be placed before Conference with housing featuring largely on the list. However it soon became clear that whilst the vast majority were expressing outright opposition and rejection of Tory policy, the resolution from Devizes was not only far more subtle but also contained an alternative and, I argued, a more socialist approach. I managed to convince two other delegates out of the forty or so involved in the discussion of the advantage and validity of the point. But the others insisted that outright opposition to Council house sales was the only viable position for the party. So, once again, the left was split on tactics and strategy.

My two colleagues and I insisted that the Devizes' resolution stood on its own and decided we should try to lobby for Trade Union support. The other two, being members of the A.E.U. and S.O.G.A.T., would approach their respective delegates and, given my rail workshop connection, suggested I take the N.U.R. and the T.G.W.U. Additionally as I had drawn up the resolution and could best explain its potential wider national implications regarding virtual nationalisation of land and Banks, then I should approach the N.U.M. who were still, in our opinion, the vanguard of the organised working class.

This I did on the Monday morning and approached Arthur Scargill outlining to him the purpose of the resolution and its potential ramifications if it were to succeed in being adopted. He patiently listened to my explanation then, with a broad grin, said "you are a devious bastard, put it to my men and if they agree we will back it". News of this, together with the other successes with S.O.G.A.T. and the A.E.U., I believe must have filtered back to the Conference Arrangements Committee because when it came to the housing debate, whilst recommending rejection of the composite, the recommendation on the Devizes resolution that was moved by myself and seconded by a man from Salford, was that it be referred to the Party E.C. where, in a typical bureaurcratic manner, whilst its referral had received great support, it was buried. The subsequent emergence of so-called "New Labour" in the mid 1990s buried forever any chance of achieving a socialist housing policy.

In the 1987–1988 period the joint approach to combat rate capping began to break down as some Metropolitan Councils began to seek accommodation with Michael Heseltine initially in respect of Liverpool and subsequently and later Manchester and Sheffield. At this time we were having some success with our "Rate Capping's Taking Your Liberty" campaign, a slogan suggested by myself which merely by the addition of "your" made use of the well known and understood working class Londoner's expression "taking a liberty" to mean any outrageous or daring manoeuvre to stretch conventionally accepted behaviour. This included such policies as the declaration of Thamesdown as a nuclear free zone. It also saw the construction and display of banners made by members of the Arts Committee in the town and the organisation of a public debate between myself and a Professor from Shrivenham Military College in one of our leisure centres which was attended by some three hundred and fifty people.

For a variety of reasons pressure was beginning to build within the Labour group, the local press and the opposition parties to seek negotiations based on Swindon's special position previously referred to as an "expanded town". The pressure within the group was primarily caused by the fear of the potential threat of surcharge which I repeatedly dismissed as I was convinced this was just a threat designed to unsettle those of a nervous disposition which was not a trait that had ever bothered me. By determined political lead and the expertise and creative thinking of an astute Borough Treasurer who was undoubtedly one of our greatest, if not the greatest, asset on the Council, we could use the surpluses generated by the Direct Labour Organisation, the transport undertaking and the "arm's length" Satman companies. However I clearly had to take account of the feelings of others. Therefore, I let it be known, that the Local Authority would be prepared to enter into discussions regarding our special position.

These discussions, however, were never to take place since with the appointment of the hard line Thatcherite, Nicholas Ridley as Secretary of State for Local Government (the member for the adjacent constituency of Cirencester) he, on a visit to Swindon, announced that in no way was the Government prepared to recognise Thamesdown's status as a special case thereby rendering any approach abortive. So instead we arranged to meet all the Council employees at a series of mass meetings, rather than just the one, in order to cut through certain inter-Union rivalries and concerns and the problem of finding a location large enough to accommodate nearly 3,000 employees.

Thus it came about that on a staggered basis and in order not to interrupt services, four separate meetings took place with three at the Wyvern Theatre and one at the Oasis Leisure Centre. Each meeting was chaired by the Trade Union side and I addressed each one explaining the Council's position regarding protection of jobs and services and I pledged the continuation of our no redundancy policy, seeking employees' assistance in ensuring the utmost efficiency, economy and effectiveness in the provision of services. I pointed out that the achievement of these aims would enable us, as an Authority, to overcome the problems being heaped onto our shoulders.

These meetings, together with the co-operation and trust they generated and achieved, led to the situation in 1990, when rate capping gave way to the Poll Tax, that Thamesdown was the only Authority to be rate capped from beginning to end of that legislation. Yet we were also the only one not to have made people redundant and had, in fact, recruited when the need arose. We had also, by independent assessment, been declared the seventh most efficient Local Authority in the country.

In February 1985 we had been described in the Labour Herald as a "beacon of socialism in Tory Wiltshire". I would contend that was indeed our position but on a wider geographical scale up until the group A.G.M. of 1990 but I will explain that contention later.

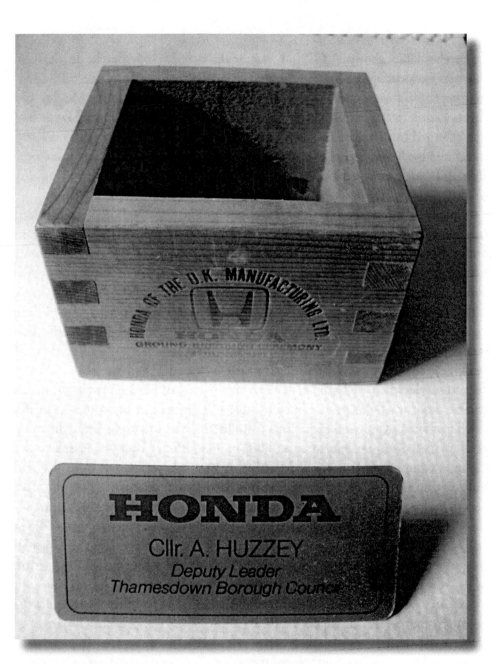

Traditional Saki drinking cup from Honda factory launch in 1984

Council Leadership, Stroke & Poll Tax

In the 1988 group A.G.M. I was again nominated for the leadership, the previous occupant having decided to step down and, in the traditional manner for Thamesdown, allowed his name to be put forward for Mayor. On this occasion however my opinion on the validity of appointing a Mayor had not changed but I raised no objection. My attempts at deleting this post and its related budgetary costs over the previous seven years had proven unacceptable and had found very little support so there was no point in raising any objections.

The so-called, or perhaps more accurately described, self-determined left, made a stupid tactical error when they nominated two of their number in opposition to my nomination when the more mellow of the two was eliminated on the first ballot. I was appointed to the position as the lesser of two evils on the second ballot.

Now, with the Government re-organising its attempts at controlling Local Government expenditure were not achieving their objectives and this was particularly true in the case of Thamesdown which appeared to them, I believe, a constant cause of annoyance since not only had we not made any cuts to services but we had, particularly in the case of leisure provision, much to the chagrin of the private sector, built a large recreation complex in the town's western expansion area. This contained a half Olympic size swimming pool, gymnasium, theatre come exhibition area, library that was leased to the County Council and an ice rink. All this had been designed in-house and built within the budget at a cost that put the private sector into despair. This centre had been built by taking out a mortgage to cover the cost of construction, the payments for which would be covered by the rents received for an adjacent shopping centre that had been built on land which the Council owned freehold. Furthermore these receipts covered a substantial proportion of the revenue costs of staffing and running the enterprise.

Having secured such expansions of provision, at no additional costs to the borough's ratepayers, the support for the Labour controlled Authority soared but we were still under considerable pressure as a result of rate capping. The resultant demands this put onto myself caused me some considerable amount of stress due to my determination to refuse the constraints the Government sought to impose.

As the rate capping legislation took hold so the pledge on which the Labour group had fought the most recent Council election in which a third of seats were contested, came under sustained pressure. We had undertaken to extend service provision by an extra £250,000 a year and this was to be shared out across all committees all of whom had entered competing bids. Competition between them was fierce and acrimonious.

The quarter of a million pound expenditure limit which the Government was imposing was completely arbitrary and took no account whatsoever of the town's continued expansion or population increase. This obviously resulted in a reduction in the Rate Support Grant paid yet such was the efficiency of our direct labour, transport, planning, car parking and recreational facilities, combined with the skill of our Treasurer, that we were able to meet our election pledges throughout the whole of the rate capping period from 1984 to 1989.

However, given all the financial pressure and competing demands, there was one thing that just could not be achieved. This was the acquisition of the Mechanics Institute which had allegedly been offered to the Council for the princely sum of £1. In my position as Chief Electrical Maintenance Foreman of the Works, together with the Mechanical and Building Maintenance Foreman, we both knew that for the past few years our budgets had been severely restrained. This meant we had been unable to carry out even the most essential work on the upkeep of this building which by then had fallen into an extreme state of degradation.

The building itself had been constructed and paid for with the active participation of the workers from the G.W.R. factory in the mid 1800s. It had been the recognised cultural and literary centre of activities having, if not the first, then one of the first, libraries and also reading rooms available for the whole populace. However when the industry was nationalised in the late 1940s the responsibility for its care and repair had come under the auspices of the Railway Board and its subsidiaries who had, for years, been neglecting those duties and were now seeking to pass them off onto the people of the town. From my own experience, coupled with that of my Maintenance Foreman colleague, we knew this would cost millions of pounds. Consequently I had no option other than to reject the £1 purchase offer.

When the site was purchased by Tarmac on the closure of the Works I endeavoured to negotiate the building's refurbishment as part of an agreed planning deal. Unfortunately, however, following their complete inspection of the building, which was very obviously riddled with both wet and dry rot, and having formerly been tied up in a similar deal with Brighton Council on the refurbishment of the Royal Pavilion, there was no way that Tarmac would entertain such an agreement.

By the end of my tenure in office the only thing I could achieve was the allocation of £125,000 to be set aside in the eventuality that this building ever became the property of the Council.

The opportunity for at least a morning's relaxation occurred in April 1988 when we received an invitation from the R.A.F. base at Lyneham for a civic visit which would include a flight in a Hercules down the Bristol Channel. I seized at the opportunity to lead a group of my fellow Council members on this trip and asked my son, Derek, if he would like to accompany me and he jumped at the chance. I had requested his company because at that time I was having some difficulty in adjusting to the so-called human insulin that I had been using for the past month.

The flight down to Lands End and back had been noisy but very pleasant. Seeing the coasts of Devon, Cornwall and Pembroke from the air gave us a whole new perspective on sights we thought we were familiar with having often walked them on ground level in the past whilst on holiday

On our return trip and as we approached Swindon, as was usual on these training flights, the load masters in the crew lowered the ramp at the rear of the plane and stretched a substantial rope net across the opening at the rear of the fuselage. On checking and receiving the go ahead to go to the net in order to take photographs I unhooked the safety harness securing me to my seat squab, normally used by parachutists, and made my way down to the rear of the plan, reasonably steadily, and took up position by the net. I was soon joined by Derek and more cautiously by most of the others in the party. With the constant throb of the turboprops and the backwash of wind from the open hatch any attempts at conversation proved nearly impossible and hand gestures had to suffice.

I shortly began to feel a bit off colour and turning to glance at the watch on my left wrist noticed that I was having difficulty in raising that arm to bring it into focus. As I recall it was about 11.45 a.m. so my first thought was that I needed to eat something so, by pointing to my mouth and making chewing movements, I indicated to Derek with my right hand that I needed some food. I then made my way steadily back up the length of the plane to where I had left my barber jacket, the pocket of which contained a slice of Joan's excellent fruit cake. Derek and one of my colleagues followed me and sat down either side of me attempting to get me to respond to their questions but, for the most part, to no avail. I ate the cake and again using hand gestures motioned to one of the crew who had previously asked me if I would like to sit in the co-pilot's seat. I asked if it would be possible for me to climb into the astrodome above the fuselage and with permission granted I made my way to that area where I remained until the plane landed.

I was the last one to disembark and one or two of my female colleagues expressed some concern at my appearance. Derek assured them, and also the R.A.F. officers who had gathered round, that I was O.K. but in need of some food. So we all retired to the Mess where a reception had been prepared but even after eating I was still struggling to speak coherently which, for me, was by no means normal.

Somewhat mystified at this turn of events and sincerely thanking our hosts, we all took our leave, boarded the coach and returned to the Civic Offices. Upon arrival I asked my shared P.A. if she could detect any difference in my normal speech or demeanour and she responded that I did sound a little slurred. Unlike myself, she was a North Londoner so was well used to my usual mode of speech but she assumed the slurring was as a result of several glasses of wine and I agreed that I had drunk at least three glasses.

In view of the fact there had been a few calls for me that morning I told her I would go to my office and deal with them. On reaching the office I sat behind my desk and reached down with my left hand to unzip my briefcase. To my confusion I could not operate it so, intrigued, lifted the briefcase, with some difficulty, onto my lap. Holding it firmly with my right hand I clamped it tightly between my knees, zip uppermost, and again tried to open the zip with my left hand but again with no success. Though I am right handed, normally, performing such simple operations with either hand was no problem.

I then tried another few simple hand manoeuvres which should have presented no problems so when even these proved difficult for me I became suspicious that these were symptoms of a stroke. I asked my P.A. to contact everyone who had left messages for me that morning and tender my apologies that I could not get back to them till the following day. I then asked her to contact Joan at the Civil Service Pension Office to tell her that I would pick her up thirty minutes' early.

It was with extreme difficulty that I managed to engage the car's reverse gear, then having to drive about half a mile to a parallel street to collect Joan. By the time I reached her office car park I would normally have been in fourth gear but my inability to use the gear box meant that I could only manage the journey in first gear. When Joan joined me at the car I asked her to take over the driving but, at that stage, withheld my suspicions about my possible stroke. Upon arriving home I went straight into the garage workshop and fashioned a sprung clamp out of two flat pieces of wood a small gate hinge, a valve spring and a three inch bolt. With this enclosed in my left hand I continually compressed the clamp exercising the affected hand, all the while attempting to sing or mumble. Sadly I had not inherited my father's singing voice but it did overcome the slurring of speech.

Later that evening, with my left hand hidden under the committee table continuously operating the clamp, I chaired a preliminary budget setting meeting of the Policy and Resources Committee. I was fully able to participate in and lead the discussions giving no-one there any cause for concern at my performance. Derek had driven me to that meeting and my Deputy had kindly given me a lift back home.

The following morning I presented myself at the doctors' surgery, having taken the bus to get me there. In the Waiting Room I encountered my daughter, Dawn, and we asked each other the purpose for our respective visits. I anticipated that, having been married some two years previously, she was about to announce that Joan and I were to become grandparents. Dawn, who was now a Senior Trauma Nursing Sister, dismissed my assumptions in that respect. I told her of my suspicions and asked her not to say anything to her mother at this stage. She told me to wait for her as my name was the first to be called.

My G.P. being away, the locum who was filling in, placed a stethoscope to my carotid arteries and told me that my suspicions were a distinct possibility. She then reached for the telephone and her note pad, wrote a letter and instructed me to present myself at the local hospital within the hour. This was at about 11.00 a.m. on a Friday morning. As I left the G.P.s office, so Dawn also emerged from an adjacent office and on hearing my news volunteered to drop me off at the hospital as she was about to start her own shift. Following an M.R.I. scan which confirmed that I had indeed experienced a mild T.I.A. (Transient Ischaemic Attack - mild stroke), I was referred to the Vascular Surgery Unit at Oxford. The appointment was made for the following Wednesday morning. I do not know if this rapid referral and subsequent vascular surgery was due to my perceived status as a local Council Leader or as a Type One diabetic of, by then, nearly forty years' duration. I trust it was the second of these but preferable that neither factor influenced the timescale. Suffice it to say that less than three weeks after the incident in the Hercules I fortunately found myself receiving the attention of another eminent Physician, Professor Peter Morris, who performed a carotid endarterectomy on the RH5 of my neck, clearing the artery of cholesterol, a flake of which had apparently previously become detached and caused the mild stroke.

At the initial consultation, Professor Morris had congratulated me on my common sense with the clamp and told me it had assisted in limiting the damage. He also congratulated me on my strict diabetic control which had sufficiently aroused the interest of and intrigued a French colleague of his who was an Anaesthetist who had come to Britain on a lecture tour. He had volunteered his services in assisting Professor Morris with my operation and in view of his colleague's international status, Professor Morris urged me to accept his offer. I duly agreed and together the three of us discussed the amount of insulin and glucose infusion I should receive during the operation and agreed that as soon as I regained consciousness then responsibility for this would again be handed back to me.

Both knowing that I was facing a major operation, Joan and I had confidentially said a temporary goodbye to each other, whilst still optimistic as to its outcome. We each gave reassurances of our enduring love and determination that this was not going to be the end of our time together. Two days later, with a vertical row of stitches running from under my chin to the base of my neck, I was wheeling a stand supporting a bag of some necessary fluid being administered to my body down the ward to the small ward kitchen to make a cup of coffee when the ward door opened and there stood Joan. She rushed forward into my outstretched arms and I just managed to steady the stand from falling with my left hand as I wrapped both arms around her. I kissed away her tears of happiness and relief whilst she attempted to make contact with my lips. When she at last succeeded we held each other in that embrace for a time before I recalled why I had started my journey down the ward and I asked her if she would like a coffee.

I had to stay in hospital for ten days during which time I underwent further MRI and ultra sound scans. I kept myself occupied by composing on paper a lecture I had been asked to do by a couple of my Council colleagues. They wanted me to address a mix of employees from W.H. Smiths, B.C.A., Reader's Digest and others connected with the print and publishing industry on the topic of a socialist's approach to Local Government. In view of the possibility of either the diabetes or the effects of the stroke forcing me to back out from this lecture I wrote it down, stencilled copies of which were handed out. This was the first and last time I ever used this practice since I had always made it a habit to respond to discussion spontaneously, usually at some length, developing the argument of the opposition, knocking it down and negating their likely response before they could even make it. One night, on the receiving end of this technique, the Director of the Arts & Recreation Committee told me, in what I assumed was meant to be complimentary, that I "was worse than a Jesuit"!

I had been told by Professor Morris that without the operation I had had to undergo I would likely to have sustained a major stroke within the next ten years and he also strongly advised that I give up smoking. For a couple of months preceding the operation I had been feeling quite lousy and in trying to rationalise why I thought there were three possible reasons for this. Firstly, prior to my marriage, Professor Lawrence had warned me that as I neared forty years duration with diabetes, which I now was, then my diabetic condition would start to go downhill. Secondly was the 25% increase in insulin strength which my limited scientific knowledge made me wonder if mass re-volume was a factor. Thirdly was the use of the so-called human insulin in place of the animal insulin I had used up until that time. There was also a fourth possible reason that struck me which, although I thought unlikely, was as a result of the air pressure changes during the flight in the Hercules. However, whatever the reason, one thing was certain, I was definitely experiencing wild fluctuations in my blood sugar levels for no apparent rational reason but deep down I felt this was due to the changes in insulin. I therefore resolved that as soon as I got home I would contact all the insulin companies I knew about to see if there were any amongst them who were still producing animal insulin.

With the assistance of a chemist who was known to Colleen and Ron who had a cleaning contract at the Burroughs and Wellcome Laboratory in which, twenty five years previously, I had been involved installing the electrics, this proved to be fruitful and he suggested I contact a colleague of his at C.P. Pharmaceuticals in North Wales. Diabetics up and down the U.K. had been informed that animal insulin was no longer available yet with a letter I requested and subsequently received I now had proof this was not the case. I immediately got a prescription from my G.P. and switched back and the problems I had been experiencing over the past three months whilst using the new human insulin promptly disappeared.

So it was that just three weeks after my operation, much to the concern of both Joan and my P.A., I duly resumed my role as Council Leader. I had picked up signs and talk of "cats and mice" which I was determined to knock on the head. There developed the usual ongoing tussle when the Community Planning Committee endeavoured to secure funding in order to retain certain areas of provision it had, despite warnings to the contrary, been foolish to set up two years previously. This had been done in the full knowledge that initial Government funding would only last for that period of time. The group agreed that if these schemes were to continue then the Committee must achieve savings elsewhere or find alternative funding as had been the case with all the other Committees.

The other main areas of contention concerned the determination to secure the maximum space possible on the site of the rail works for employment provision. Tarmac, the development company who had purchased the site, wanted to develop it as a shopping area with a limited housing element. However it was felt that another shopping development here would threaten the Council's main asset, i.e. the Brunel Shopping Centre. So in order to enhance the Council's negotiating position I instructed the Planning Officers to seek Preservation Orders on as many of the site's buildings as possible. When subsequently granted these covered approximately sixty percent of the site to the east of Rodbourne Road and everything to the west with the exception of the Pattern Store and weighbridge which was flattened.

Another area of contention, with both the Government and a Consortium of developers, was on the northern periphery of the town where the Council were fighting to prevent a 16,000 house development. The Council had initially refused consent for successive planning applications each of which had failed to meet our genuine concerns with regard to the provision of adequate infrastructure, schools, medical and social facilities, etc. Unfortunately the Government Inspector came down on the side of the developers but indicated the development could only go ahead if financial agreement regarding infrastructure provision could be reached between Wiltshire County Council, Thamesdown Borough Council and the Development Consortium. The initial offer on the table was £11 million which we considered to be grossly inadequate. However the Tory controlled County Council were by no means as resolute as ourselves and the negotiations became very protracted. Eventually, by dint of argument in early 1989, came the threat of Wiltshire County Council either pulling out of the discussions or reaching a separate agreement.

December 1988 had, however, been an auspicious month. The annual Audit Commission report carried out that year by the independent auditor, Arthur Young on the criteria "value for money" had, as it had in previous years, been consistently judged a well managed Authority. This year, the fourth since we had been rate capped, and despite the Government's endeavours, Thamesdown had neither cut its services nor declared any redundancies. We achieved, and I quote, "congratulations are in order, particularly when compared with other authorities". This praise came just days after the then Secretary of State for Local Government, Nicholas Ridley, had condemned us for "bad expensive delivery of services". This demonstrated not only the rage of the Government at its failure to quell a successful Labour controlled Authority, but also its failure to read the reports which it had itself commissioned.

Further good news came that month when we completed negotiations with the Nationwide for its relocation to a site on the southern edge of the town with a promised four hundred clerical jobs on completion. Additionally, it was agreed that only local labour would be utilised in the construction of the £50 million development.

Furthermore Motorola announced its intention to set up a £20 million base on the Council owned site at Blagrove with a further three hundred jobs.

On the 20th December 1988 an amusing list appeared in the local press which caused those closest to me, i.e. family and Council officers, some hilarity. It was headed "Christmas List" and against my name was a suggested A-Z of City of London finance deals, whilst against the name of my main critic had been placed a "Tony Huzzey" dart board and, obviously, in the eyes of the media, such was our domination of the Council and electorate support that the list read Thamesdown Council an opposition.

Finally, I received a request from the Wilshire Gazette & Herald Business Section to write an article headed "Business and Industry" which would be syndicated nationally for Kemsley Press.

On a more personal front, in 1985, after we had celebrated our twenty fifth wedding anniversary, an event that deeply affected myself and Joan occurred. We still both felt exactly the same about each other as we had on that day twenty five years earlier only more so than ever. There had, however, been developments closer to home that had been causing me great concern and this was in relation to Joan's health. As was her usual habit when I enquired of her what was wrong, she just dismissed my persistent questioning. However, one night, during our usual pre-coital embraces, she pushed my hand away from her left breast and at last admitted she was worried about a possible lump that she had detected. I touched the area and confirmed there was indeed a hard lump there which felt about the size of a marble and she finally agreed to my repeated urges to see the G.P. I must admit that until she had drawn my attention to the exact location of this lump I had noticed any changes to my beautiful wife's glorious figure during our frequent love making but it was now determined that this discovery should be swiftly sorted.

The G.P. subsequently referred Joan to the hospital to see the relevant Consultant which caused her some initial concern. This turned to consternation when, on entering his office and following his examination of her remarked that he had recognised her name but had not realised she was my wife. On seeing Joan's quizzical expression to this he told her not to worry it was just that he had met me some years ago when the local branch of the B.D.A. had been established. He told her that his own son was a Type One diabetic and that I had been a great encouragement to him especially when I had reassured his wife that their son, like myself, could also lead a good life despite the condition.

He told Joan that he would perform a lumpectomy and if the lump proved to be a cyst or benign then it would be removed but if it was malignant then it may be necessary for her to undergo a course of radiotherapy. He told her not to worry and that he would operate as soon as possible.

As per the usual three year requirement for Type One diabetics, in that September I had had to re-apply for my driving licence. However, much to my surprise, on this occasion I was issued with a licence that was not due to expire until my seventy fourth birthday.

For the most part Joan, bless her, was determined to carry on as usual and now, since she had assumed the main driving role, was equally determined to drive herself to Oxford for the radiotherapy treatment despite the caution she had been advised to adopt by one of her work colleagues who was also a close neighbour who had herself undergone the same treatment. So, after her first treatment, she reluctantly accepted that I should drive on the return journey. I could see that in addition to the discomfort the procedure caused her she was also far more nervous than she had ever been over the past thirty years when occupying the front passenger seat. We followed that same pattern right up to the end of her treatment cycle.

At around that time Joan was also concerned, as I was, with regard to a symptom I had been developing which that nearly forty years earlier Dr Lawrence had cautioned me about. I now had virtually no sign of the onset of a hypo and had, as always, tried to carry on as normal. It was invariably only a blood test, which were now standard, that would reveal whether or not I was actually experiencing a hypo or not. Neither Joan nor the children were happy with this situation and under no circumstances would the medics accept that it did not affect my performance. That is until one day in the mid 1990s when, following my expressed desire to seek a second opinion, my G.P. secured an appointment for me to see Professor Stephanie Amiel who now occupied Dr Lawrence's chair at King's College Hospital.

It was now some forty years since I had last seen the man himself and the clinic had certainly changed over that time. Now, on entering, an immediate blood sample was taken and evaluated in the laboratory attached. I had been having discussions with Professor Amiel for about thirty minutes when suddenly the door opened and a nurse entered bearing a glass of glucose which she handed to me with instructions to drink it. I placed it on the desk in front of me and said "no thank you". When the alarmed nurse revealed my blood test results had registered 1.8 mml the Professor asked me what I would normally do. I responded that I would usually eat the sandwich which I always carried in my pocket and proceeded to do just that much to the amazement of the nurse who was still present. Professor Amiel assured the concerned nurse that after having diabetes now for forty years I knew what I was doing. She later assured me that my behaviour and contribution to the discussion had indeed been rational and, bearing in mind my blood sugar levels, I had in no way displayed any intellectual impairment. However, in view of the fact that I had now experienced two mild strokes I should quadruple my Aspirin dose to 300 mg daily. She went on to say that I was the personification of the validity of Dr Lawrence's methods of diabetic control which were based on strict carbohydrate control intake.

Some ten years later, during the late 1990s, the B.D.A. put out an appeal for the four hundred or so of its members who had survived for nearly fifty years with the condition to contact them. They wanted us to participate in a scientific analysis entitled "The Golden Years" and so I duly became a participant in this research project, the results of which were, I thought, of great significance. It ultimately emerged that amongst all the participants there were no cases of kidney disease, no amputees, no obesity and no cases of blindness although the majority did have some degree of retinopathy which had required minor laser treatment. So it was that none of us had any of the symptoms or effects of uncontrolled diabetes. The one thing we all had in common was that we had all been taught, and continued to follow, strict carbohydrate control.

To return to the political situation then pertaining in Thamesdown, in 1989 the Tory Government had decided nationally to supersede rate capping which had not achieved the degree of control of Local Government expenditure it had been required to do. This was most certainly the case in Thamesdown which had become the only non-Metropolitan borough to be rate capped every year of the five year duration of that legislation. Indeed, such had been our resistance and continued expansion of services, despite the restrictions placed on us, that the electorate were, it seemed, thoroughly behind us having reduced the Tory element on the Council to a mere twelve in number. The replacement legislation was somewhat erroneously called the Community Charge but was rapidly and correctly referred to as the Poll Tax, the first time such a measure had been introduced since the peasants' revolt in 1381 and the resulting uproar was almost as great as that in the fourteenth century.

In Thamesdown this initially presented itself on the night of the Policy and Resources Committee budget setting meeting when, by careful accounting and maximum utilisation of all available resources, we managed to bring forward a proposed budget that would protect all existing services and personnel but would be just marginally below the Government's £15 million limit that would subject non-Metropolitan Councils to potential capping, in view of the fact that that would require a Poll Tax precept of £336, which exceeded the Government's purely hypothetical figure of £238. As the overall potential cap was set at £15 million, the Borough Solicitor, Treasurer and myself, were agreed we could challenge any cap at a judicial review if necessary. However I had some difficulty persuading the group of this potential course of action since the fear of surcharge again seized quite a high percentage of them and the self declared left were, as usual, calling for outright refusal to set a figure at all despite knowing full well that such a move would make it impossible for the Council to operate with the inevitable complete collapse of both services and employment of staff. Nevertheless they persisted in that demand.

On the night of the Policy and Resources Committee meeting I arranged for this to take place in the Chamber rather than the usual Committee Room in order to facilitate maximum public access and also arranged for a P.A. system to be installed. There were clear indications there would be a sizeable number of people wishing to hear the discussions that night. I arrived at approximately 6.45 p.m. in time for the meeting which was due to start at 7.00 p.m. and I made my way through a large crowd that was gathered in the parking area and on the steps of the Civic Offices. There were many faces that I recognised amongst the throng and I found myself explaining the position to all that would listen which, with very few exceptions, met with a favourable response. Much to my surprise there were about a dozen police officers standing at the top of the steps barring entry to the doors and it was with some difficulty that I managed to persuade them to let me enter the building but that was only after the Council's doorkeeper confirmed my identity. I was then informed that the public gallery was full and the police had been instructed by their Commander not to allow further admissions. Before I went inside to chair the meeting I drew to the attention of those closest to me that there was a P.A. system installed.

Some ten minutes into proceedings the Chamber doors suddenly burst open and a large number of people surged into the Chamber, many of them flowing down the left hand aisle where their progress was impeded by a tripod upon which was mounted a T.V. camera and its accompanying crew. Others dashed along the front to use the right hand aisle which was similarly occupied by press reporters with still more people leaping onto the desk-type shelves behind which sat the Lay Councillors and senior officers. People made their way, shelf by shelf, to the back of the Chamber beneath the Public Gallery to occupy the space behind the rear row of seats which were already full.

As Council Leader I sat in my usual seat on the dias in front of the Chamber, with the other seats being occupied by the rest of the committee, Chairs and Directors of the Council, i.e. Borough Treasurer, Housing, Arts & Recreation, Planning & Environmental Services. I was then approached by the senior police officer who enquired if I wanted them to clear the Chamber to which I emphatically responded that I did not. My response was somewhat to the dissatisfaction of the Chief Executive and also, judging by the look of alarm on their faces, to the consternation of my assembled colleagues. This was amidst shouts of "resign" from the more vociferous of those in the Public Gallery to which I responded that was exactly what Thatcher had been trying to make us do for the past five years but we had resisted her efforts throughout that period and had no intention of complying now. I endeavoured to make the most of the opportunity to put forward the case against the iniquity of the Poll Tax and the value to the citizens of comprehensive public services supplied through the means of democratically elected and resourced Councils participating fully with their electorate in both implementation and administration which we had established and intended to continue to enhance.

It was around this time, during the lunch break at one of the regular meetings of the rate capped Authorities, that Ken Livingstone, the leader of the Greater London Council, had revealed to me that considering the difference between our respective populations and revenue income, Thamesdown had equalled, if not exceeded, the achievements of the G.L.C. during the period of rate capping with regard to the provision of services.

In order to continue that process no other option was available to us other than, despite our opposition in principle to the legislation, to set a figure to enable the Council to continue to exist. A spokesman for the protesters asked if he could have the microphone to address the meeting. He struck me as being one of the more rational of those clamouring at the front of the dias so I told him that I would allow him two minutes in which to speak. He gave assurances that he would return the microphone at the end of his allotted two minutes.

So I vacated the dias and walked over to him where he was located in the middle of the throng of people and handed him the microphone. After indicating to him that his two minutes were up he did indeed honour his side of the agreement and went to hand the microphone back to me. By this time, however, Council agendas were being torn up or thrown around the room by many of the people gathered there. Unfortunately, whatever the cause, the

head of the microphone was knocked off and as I stooped to retrieve it someone started to beat me about the head and shoulders using a rolled up agenda.

I thought this had now gone far enough so I stepped forward to the front
of the assembled committee members occupying the front row of seats and
moved the vote to set the Council Tax. I raised my arm and asked all in favour
to do likewise.

Thus passed the most distasteful experience of my period serving on Swindon Council.

Much to my distress I had now become the instrument through which the
Council had had to implement a thoroughly iniquitous and unjust taxation
on the people of Swindon, a town that twenty nine years earlier, had become
my home. This had to be done in order to keep in operation a Local Authority that had, I believed, up to that point, achieved much for its population.

As I left the Chamber headed for my office amidst shouts of "Judas" and
"traitor" I felt that I desperately needed a drink. Surprisingly I was feeling
completely calm although somewhat annoyed. The meeting that night should
have been an opportunity to present a reasoned and justified condemnation of
this tax which was being imposed on people without any fair process whatsoever in ascertaining their ability to pay. The majority who had come together
that night to make a fair and peaceful protest had been sabotaged by a minority of idiots who had sought to gain some cheap political advantage from the
fully justified concerns of the people of Thamesdown.

However there were some surprises yet in store, the first of which occurred
the following weekend when I learned that the media description of the
so-called "riot and invasion of Thamesdown's Council Chamber" had received
widespread coverage not only on British T.V. but also much further abroad.
My daughter's partner was, at that time, serving with the R.A.F. at a base on
the Belgium and West German border where the T.V. coverage had also been
screened and he passed on to her some complimentary comments regarding
my conduct. Likewise, the friend of one of my colleagues who was in Honk
Kong had received a telephone call from him similarly complimenting me on
my performance that night.

The other surprise was a request that I should be present at the BBC's
Bristol studio the following week to take part in a Newsnight Special live
debate. This I agreed to do provided my travelling expenses were met and I
was supplied with a sandwich. So it was the following week, having driven
down to Bristol on my way to the BBC studio, I found myself confronted by a
large crowd of people demonstrating outside Bristol Town Hall. The placards
they were carrying contained angry protestations against the Poll Tax. As I

came to a halt behind another car the crowd started milling around us and my attention was drawn to a man who was rapping on my window which, in some trepidation, I lowered a few inches. The man drew his head level with mine and asked me if I was the man from Swindon. When I replied that I was he asked me where I was going and on receipt of my response he said he would ensure that I got through the crowd. Firstly, however, he asked me why I, a self declared socialist, was driving a pale blue Volkswagen. I responded that if his knowledge of politics was based on a liking of colour then whilst mine was red with strong green undertones, there was no way I would choose either as a car colour. I advertised my politics by what I said and did and I suggested that he did the same. With that rebuke he grinned and said that perhaps he had better start now then and walking into the throng of people he started yelling for them to make way and that I was one of them. So I progressed until we came to a police cordon where I had to persuade a Police Inspector to allow me to proceed to the T.V. studio.

Upon arrival I was given a sandwich and a cup of coffee and after some twenty minutes of uncertainty it was finally confirmed that due to a technical hitch we would be unable to link with the Bristol studio. I was understandably annoyed at this but duly made my, via back streets, to the M4 and hence back home.

A week or so later, despite protests from both the anti tax demonstrators, organisers and some of our group members, the Mayor, who was also Chair, decided that the next full Council/Poll Tax ratification meeting would be held in the Council Chamber as usual and not in a larger venue, i.e. a leisure centre, a decision I was in full agreement with. He did, however, also make another decision which I was not in favour of and that was, in addition to requesting police attendance, we should also hire a private security force inside the building to ensure there was no repetition of the scenario of the previous meeting when the main doors were burst in and the Chamber was invaded by hoards of concerned residents.

In the event, this meeting passed off much more calmly although there was still a large mass of protestors outside the building. Unlike most of the other Councillors I had again entered the building by the front doors threading my way through the crowd gathered outside. Many of those people present made it clear that they had had no part in the demonstration of the week before and that their lobby then had been usurped by extreme left and right wing elements. They were, however, genuinely concerned at the inequalities obviously rampant in the imposition of this tax which was based on the individual rather than the property and gave no consideration whatsoever of people's ability to pay. Large numbers of these people had one or more young adults still living at home who now, with the fall in employment, which in the Thatcher years had become rampant, annual rates for many of them would quadruple. Statistics at that time showed there were at least three family members within the average family who were unemployed. In addition people were also concerned at the potential loss of Council services which they had come to appreciate to an even greater degree in the ten years of Labour's control of the Council. It was also made clear that they did not hold Local Authorities responsible for this tax, at least not those controlled by the Liberals or Labour. Nevertheless they were intent on expressing their concern and discontent which was subsequently made very clear as I saw later from a video recording of the proceedings when an effigy of Mrs Thatcher had been hung on a long pole and then, to loud cheers, set alight.

This time, inside the Council Chamber we received only perfunctory interjections from the gallery which was again filled to capacity. What comments did come from that quarter were directed, in the main, at the Tories, aside from one or two of the self proclaimed left grandstanding which, much to their surprise, received a very muted response.

So the Poll Tax was set and my attention was then shifted since I had made it clear I did not intend to seek re-election in 1992 by which time I would have served three complete terms. That, together with the fact that the twenty first century was now less than ten years off, our attention should be focused on forward planning. I therefore arranged for a full day brain storming session to be attended by the Committee Chairs, the Directors of those areas the Committees covered, plus the Head of Personnel, the Treasurer, Solicitor, Chief Executive and myself. The venue for this was Urchfont Manor.

The main concern, that I expressed, and which indeed was also shared by the town's inhabitants, was one that had become increasingly clear to officers and members alike over the course of the preceding decade. This was in relation to the continuing expansion of Swindon and despite the difficulties that would inevitably arise I secured agreement that we should attempt to place a periphery beyond which development would be prohibited. This was adopted by the full Council prior to May of that year when Joan and I were scheduled to take a much needed holiday.

Having decided we would use this opportunity to use our rail passes we approached the man who organised trips for existing and former rail workers to find out what was on offer. Joan did not fancy a cross Canada rail trip as it would involve flying there and back which made her very nervous. Another option we were both agreed upon was a trip to Norway, part of which would be by ship from Oslo to Flam up the coastal line. This had an attraction for me as in the mid 1950s, when my parents had first acquired a television, I watched a programme, made in black and white of course, that Cliff Mitchelmore had made of the journey up the Norwegian coast that had really stuck in my memory. I assured Joan this would be similar, but potentially even more spectacular, than our trip through Scotland which we had both loved. This trip only being available during the first week of May we duly made our booking although it had meant that I would miss the group A.G.M. but I was not unduly concerned about that. This time I was putting Joan and myself first.

In late 1989 I had started working in a local factory that produced cold cabinets for Sainsbury. They employed about four hundred workers in all but were in need of a second electrician. My counterpart had also served in the rail works and we had spent some time together when he was an apprentice so we already knew each other.

It soon became clear to me that working for this company did not place me in a very good situation as the amount of work currently available was clearly not enough to last for the next six months. The management, however, were confident that things would pick up but given the state of the economy at that time I was extremely dubious, particularly as both the T&G and A.E.U. stewards had informed me that the company were not very forthcoming with any detailed information in that regard. So, using my contacts, I obtained detailed reports about the company's financial position from Companies House and duly made these available to the stewards and their respective area officials. The telephone on the shop floor was tied up every morning at the 10.00 a.m. tea break by my P.A. ringing in and checking things out with me, much to the amusement of my colleagues who often observed that I was running an organisation of that size over the telephone yet the managers there could not even organise the flow from fifty yards away.

In view of the fact that I was going to miss the A.G.M. I decided to circulate a letter to the sitting Labour Councillors and also those that were standing for election that year indicating that if they were satisfied with my current working status and also my performance on the Council since my operation then I was still capable of performing adequately as Leader. If the general consensus was in agreement then I was prepared to continue in this position but that I had resolved not to seek re-election in 1992.

Having said that, however, I was by now somewhat dubious about my abilities to continue working at my trade since following my stroke, I seemed to have lost the ability to reverse things through one 180° in my mind and I was also losing the ability of reading drawings and other aspects essential to my trade.

My fellow spark pointed out to me one morning a potential fault on a cabinet I had been working on. I thanked him for this and asked him if he would mind keeping an eye on me and confided to him that I would probably quit when I returned from holiday since there was no way I was going to risk putting anyone in danger of receiving an electric shock from a cabinet I had made. He assured me that nothing he had seen of my work had been anywhere near that serious. Nevertheless I could not ignore my niggling and increasing concern about my diminishing capability to carry out my trade.

On the start of our holiday, as the train pulled into Durham, I was once again struck with the shear majesty of the cathedral as it came into view. I had first explored this beautiful building with Joan in 1959 when she had taken me up north to introduce me to her relatives. However, of some concern to us was the fact that the train was running about half an hour late and we were worried that we were going to miss the boat. In the event, however, we made it up the gangplank by the skin of our teeth. As we left the Tyne Joan told me of the joys of Rocar and her visits there with her grandparents as a youngster during the war years.

The next morning, as we passed the midway point between Newcastle and Oslo, our attention was drawn by the tannoy to the presence of a whale some-way off. It remained in sight for at least twenty minutes or so and was quite an exciting experience.

That first night was spent on the ship in Oslo harbour, a place we decided we would like to see more of when we departed from there in a fortnight's time. The following day we went ashore at Bergen where we were very impressed with the medieval wooden constructions. The other thing that amazed us was the fantastic variety of fish available on the keyside market and the beauty of the reflections in the fjords of the surrounding mountains and countryside along the coast.

That holiday gave us both a chance to wind down from all the stress and trauma of the preceding months, particularly our concerns with regard to Joan's health. This was aided in no small measure by the breathtaking scenery and weather although it was incongruous in the extreme. One day, in brilliant sunshine, whilst on a coach trip and travelling alongside a precipice, the driver pulled over in order to allow us to gaze down on the small frozen lakes hundreds of feet below. Being dressed in a tee shirt and shorts and wearing my walking boots, I took the opportunity to walk a hundred yards back up the road so that Joan could take a photograph of me standing with snow piled at least forty feet high on either side of the road. This, I felt, really demonstrated our country's inability to cope with the effects of winter on our own infrastructure for this was early May!

The only problem we experienced on that holiday was at meal times. The spread on the smörgåsbord[7] table was incredible yet it was all too often the case that when we, in the last one third of the queue, reached the front the metre long salmon was reduced to a mere skeleton and the shrimp and meat trays would frequently be empty. It amazed us that the dozen or so, mainly British, pensioners in front of us could eat so much. It was after all nearly fifty years since the end of food rationing and this greed disgusted the pair of us.

The Norwegian staff were utterly perplexed when, on a number of occasions due to the dictates of my diabetes, we had to appeal for extra food. So thereafter, for both the lunch and evening meals, they kindly put food aside for Joan and myself. Breakfast however was not a problem we both normally ate cereal of one kind or another which, compared to the amount and variety of protein on offer, seemed to be low on everyone else's agenda.

As the holiday came to an end and we were looking out on Norway's pleasant countryside having returned to Oslo from Flam by train, our thoughts turned to home and what possible surprises may await us there. One thing which I fully expected but which Joan thought unlikely was that I was no longer Leader of the Council. This was confirmed by Derek who collected us at Swindon station when asked by Joan "what was new?" Her response to this was much harsher than mine and not at all complimentary to my fellow group members.

---

7 * Scandinavian buffet style meal with multiple dishes of various food originated in Sweden.

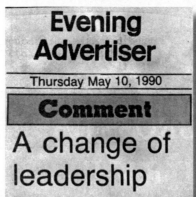

Evening Advertiser

Thursday May 10, 1990

Comment

A change of leadership

Labour politics in Swindon owes a lot to Councillor Tony Huzzey, who has been replaced as Leader of Thamesdown Borough Council. Unlike the high profile largely ceremonial position of Mayor, the job of leader of the majority group, which carries with it the chairmanship of the powerful policy and resources committee, is one calling for supreme political skill and frenetic behind-the-scenes activity.

Mr Huzzey did not want to give up the job, but his health is such that his colleagues felt he was unable to perform at the consistently high level which two weeks ago helped Labour to secure a stronger grip on the borough than it has ever enjoyed before.

Skill and judgment

The fact that the party's vote in the local elections on a 40 per cent turnout was only 2,000 short of the performance at the General Election on a 70 per cent poll can be partly attributed to the performance of the council, and ultimately its leader.

It has not been an easy time for councils just lately, particularly those of a political persuasion different from that pertaining in Whitehall, and it has needed a great deal of skill and political judgment to ensure the standard of services remain acceptable, and even improve.

Under Tony Huzzey's leadership Thamesdown has continued its dramatic growth and his shrewd financial stewardship has seen the end of the burden of rate or poll tax capping without a reduction in services.

Tony Huzzey has left the borough in a sound condition, and it is to be hoped that his colleagues will recognise this in the year ahead.

His successor has a hard act to follow.

Leader article in Swindon Advertiser May 10 1990

••• 217 •••

Flat 42, The Circle
Pinehurst.
Thursday.

Dear Cls. Huzzey.
     Your
I have today read article in the
Thameshaven News regarding 'Rate
Capping' and am more convinced than
ever that councils should allowed
to run their own affairs.

  The government has enough troubles
nationally without interfering with
local matters. If we have confidence
to elect men to act for us, then they
should be allowed to act as they
think fit in the interest of the entire
community. I for one do not wish
to see services reduced in any way, as
many pensioners, worse off than myself,
may suffer.

  I hope that on March 7th the Council
will stand firm, against Rate
Capping.
     Yours faithfully
     Hubert Beckett,
    (Pensioner: 77 yrs).
         P.T.O.

Congratulations and thanks for all
that is being done for the elderly.

Above and right: Letters of appreciation re stance on Poll Tax

692603 153, Okus Road,
Swindon.
SN1 4JY
6 - 3 - 90

Dear Tony,

In common with many Swindon residents I have followed with interest the reports about the Poll Tax protests. I have heard you and others quoted in the Press and heard you speak on television. I sympathise with the problems and criticisms you are currently facing in implementing an iniquitous tax.

Jim D'Avila was, I know, quoted as saying you displayed "a lot of bottle" in your handling of recent events. I'd like you to know that I and many many others endorse that statement entirely. You displayed a whole crate of it! You have, I believe, also shown, as always, an equally important quality which will get you through this crisis. That is complete integrity. Keep it up. You are doing an excellent job in impossible circumstances.

Yours sincerely,

Ken Jolly.

Commemorative paperweight presented to me by Swindon Enterprise
Trust to mark my term as Governor

End of my Working Life and Joan's Declining Health

On the following Monday morning I arrived at work and handed in my notice. I was however asked if I would work out the week and, given my previous experience as Maintenance Foreman in the rail works, requested to check out a bending machine which had been causing a great deal of problems with the company's production schedules. I agreed to this on the proviso that I would endeavour to identify and if possible isolate or circumvent the fault but if it resulted in awaiting the acquisition of replacement components then the end of the week was my limit.

The machine's operators, who were around the same age as myself, gave me a breakdown of the problems being experienced. The machine itself was easily older than any of us and I soon established the probable cause of the problem and my suspicions were confirmed when I stripped down the controller and examined the segments. From my rail works days I knew by experience that the chances of obtaining replacement parts was extremely unlikely, even if the machine's manufacturer was still trading. Commissioning replacement segments and contacts would potentially not only be expensive but also difficult and time consuming. I duly relayed this information to the manager and recommended serious thought be given into looking for a more modern replacement as in the longer term that would be far more economically viable.

So it was that at the end of that week, on the Friday afternoon, I bid farewell to my work mates. I also did something I had previously been determined never to entertain, having I suppose, refused to accept the fact. I had to face up to the fact that I was disabled now. Following the disconcerting loss of the 180° element I had come to the conclusion that I should perhaps accept this fact if I wanted to continue working. So I became the holder of a green card.

The question of continued work, however, was taken out of my hands. The following Monday when I attended the doctors' surgery to get a prescription my G.P., Peter, whom I had known now for thirty years, asked me what was the matter during the course of our discussion as I seemed to be on edge. I told him that I was due to attend a meeting to which he replied that he was under the impression that I had finished with all that, meaning the Council. I assured him that was indeed the case but the meeting was with the Ministry of Labour to sign on! He looked somewhat startled at this then looked me straight in the eye and said "Tony, you have been diabetic since you were twelve; you have been working since you were fifteen; you have done your share. It is about time that you took account of your own situation. You have had a stroke and a serious operation and your condition is ongoing. You are not going to like it but in my opinion you are no longer fit enough for work and I am signing you off so forget about signing on!"

Thus ended my working life. When I told Joan about this her immediate reaction was "that's a load off my mind, I've been of the same opinion for some time". So we both made the necessary adjustments in our life and now only having two years left to pay on the mortgage I decided to pay that off thereby making a saving on the mortgage protection policy which, due to my diabetes, had been subject to a 40% loading. I was also entitled to take a reduced pension at age 50 from the now defunct rail works which, even though I would now be in receipt of sickness benefit too, things were still going to be financially tight for us.

It was about a year or so after this that my attention was drawn to an article in the Diabetic Association journal, "Balance" about the parents of an eleven year old diabetic receiving Disability Living Allowance in respect of their child's condition. This took me aback somewhat because even from the age of twelve, when I had first been diagnosed, I had never considered myself to be disabled and indeed still could not. I failed to comprehend why any parent would willingly place their child in this category or imprint upon their child that diabetes was a disability. The condition had never prevented me from doing anything I wanted to do. It just taught me to understand the way my body works, what can go wrong and how to deal with it if it should.

Nevertheless, in 1992, in view of our now restrained financial circumstances, I decided to apply for this benefit for which I was turned down. Having now had the condition for forty two years and since it was a benefit being paid to the parents of the child in the article I had read, I went ahead and appealed this decision in full anticipation of an opportunity for a lively discussion on the ambiguity of the situation. This, however, proved not to be necessary. Some years before I had been a member of the committee which gave rise to the establishment of the Thamesdown Law Centre, part of whose remit it was to cover welfare benefits. They managed to obtain the guidelines which governed the decision making process of the Disability Living Allowance adjudicators and, as revealed in their decision in relation to myself, this proved they were in direct contradiction of their own guidelines. So the Law Centre sent a letter to them on my behalf detailing the relevant clause in this regard. This had the effect of a rapid reversal of the D.L.A.'s previous decision to refuse me this benefit and I duly received a back-dated payment from the date of my original application. However now, some eighteen years later, after that original decision despite the fact that the passage of time has taken its inevitable toll, their assessment of my condition in relation to care and mobility remains unchanged which is, I feel, ridiculous. However that is bureaucracy for you.

The 1990s, as a decade, brought about many emotional blows to Joan and myself. The fist of these was the loss of her father, Albert, and then, a year later, the circumstances around the tragic birth of our first grandchild. From the onset of her pregnancy Dawn had made the medics aware of the incidence of spina bifida in the family and that her first cousin was a victim of this condition. From her scans however, nothing was revealed to her that her baby may also have the condition which later proved to be a gross error. Her baby had, in fact, a much more severe case of spina bifida than her cousin and died in her arms twenty minutes after the birth. As can be imagined we were all utterly devastated.

Two years later Dawn successfully gave birth to our grandson, Alex, in whom we all delighted. However, some months later, fate again dealt us a blow when my father succumbed to prostrate cancer. Then, another two years on, came the greatest shock of all when our brother-in-law, Ron, on returning from a weekend caravanning with Colleen, and after unlocking the front door of their house pushed it open and collapsed into the passage, dying instantly with a heart attack. He was the youngest of the four of us.

The final blow came, again after a two year gap. Joan and I were on another camping holiday, the approximate location of which Dawn had given Colleen who was trying to contact me. By a process of elimination she was finally able to get a message to me to contact her. When I did she told me that our mother had died. There were also other, but less disturbing blows in the 1990s which really was a very difficult decade for us.

In the mid 1980s, when Dawn left us to get married, we had experienced the first elements of "empty nest syndrome". On the plus side however she was at least still living in Swindon and was now Sister in charge of the Orthopaedic and Trauma recovery wards at the Princess Margaret Hospital and also Deputy Head of Nursing.

Her brother, Derek, who had completed his apprenticeship with an H.N.C. in engineering, had been encouraged to continue with his studies by his employer. So, on day release, he attended Berks University and his mother and I took great delight in seeing him in cap and gown receiving his

BSc Honours Degree in Engineering and Production Technology. Our children had done us proud. A year or so earlier Derek had also bought a two bedroom house in Swindon which meant that Joan and I now occupied our house alone.

In the mid 1980s, after perusing "Which" magazine and a number of other car reviews, I passed the Renault 4 onto Derek. After I had played one dealer off against another I then purchased a new Volkswagon Polo at £650 below the list price. With that saving, together with what we had received for the sale of the trailer tent, we also acquired a collapsible caravan.

Just prior to Christmas in 1992, whilst watching the evening news, I suddenly became aware that I could not see out of my right eye. Obviously somewhat alarmed for several minutes I tried various manoeuvres like covering my left eye, etc., which indeed confirmed that my right eye was not functioning. With my background knowledge of diabetes, my first thought was that a blood vessel in my retina had burst. So I gingerly made my way upstairs to find Joan who was making herself ready to go out with her workmates for a meal. I asked her if she could see any discolouration in my eye which proved not to be the case. Despite her protests I insisted that she did not change her plans and still go out with her friends.

Since there was no obvious apparent problem I would arrange to see the Ophthalmologist whom I had seen previously following some minor laser treatment on that eye. She had assured me at that time that I had the finest set of eyes she had ever seen in any diabetic ever referred to her but in the event of any problems arising in the future then I should have no hesitation in contacting her again.

The following morning I presented myself at the clinic where, some thirty minutes later following a very thorough examination, the Ophthalmologist emerged into the corridor where I was now sitting reading and informed me that she could find nothing to cause her to change her original opinion. The only logical explanation she could give, in light of my previous medical history, was that I had perhaps experienced a second minor stroke but from her tests everything now seemed to be OK, as the reading charts confirmed. She once again congratulated me on my adherence to my strict diabetes control and was the first of a number of medics who have subsequently told me that I appear to be indestructible.

With it now being just the two of us and having obtained a more combined camping unit that was much more comfortable than the previous one Joan and I spent most weekends away although closer to home than before. A particular favourite location was the Malverns. One morning whilst staying on a site some two miles outside the town of Great Malvern, we decided to walk into town with the intention of buying some milk prior to climbing up to the ridge and walking the range. It being a Saturday morning the road through the town was busy and we were continuously crossing and re-crossing it through moving traffic as I sought a public toilet which I badly needed. I was also seeking a shop to buy a small bar of fruit and nut chocolate.

When I eventually located one we had by that time reached the park at the base of the hills where we located a toilet block. I removed the haversack I was carrying and passed it to Joan suggesting she sit on the bench that was located a few yards off and get out the lunch. I would join her when I had visited the toilet. This I did, not yet having eaten the chocolate. When I joined her the first thing I did was to do a blood test which revealed a BM of 0.8. According to medical science I should have been unconscious on the floor yet only moments before I had been negotiating my way through pedestrian and motor traffic with no bother whatsoever. I had had the metre checked so I knew the reading to be accurate. We walked the Mendip range that afternoon and it was a really nice day.

The one problem that weekend was in connection with erecting the collapsible caravan. The procedure for this was to first bring the front and back walls to the vertical position which then uncovered the end wall and roof sections. These were hinged in the centre. The left end then had to be brought to the vertical and secured to the front and rear walls. Then, like the flap of an envelope, the hinged half roof section had to be brought up and across. The exercise then had to be repeated on the right hand end and the two roof sections locked together so securing the whole unit.

On a calm day, this process could be completed in less than five minutes but if the weather was breezy this could make things difficult, if not dangerous because at the point of unfolding the second section of roof into position it meant that the top of my head was just three inches above the surrounding walls. On a number of occasions the wind lifted the right hand roof section out of my grasp only moments later for it to slam violently down again on the top of my head. On the first few occasions this happened it caused us both some amusement albeit it also caused me to utter a string of expletives. However on one occasion when we were holidaying on Exmoor, it caught me such a clout that it I was momentarily knocked out, much to Joan's concern.

During this period a number of strange incidents also occurred which caused me to obtain a number of scientific research papers on the long term implication of diabetes on the central nervous system, since I was experiencing an involuntary contraction of my facial muscles, particularly round the eyes and mouth. These occurred irrespective of whether my blood sugar levels were high, low or normal, but would invariably be more acute soon after eating or injecting insulin. So, following my established work study and electrical backgrounds, I started to record all relevant information onto detailed charts which I took with me to appointments with my then Diabetic Consultant with whom I had somewhat guarded relationship. He believed that my approach to my condition was outdated and I, in my turn, believed that he was perhaps prepared to ignore my forty odd years' experience of living with the condition.

On one such appointment in 1992 Joan had, for the first time ever, attended an appointment with me. The Consultant had asked if I was still driving to which I responded that I was but only on seldom occasions. He then turned to Joan and asked her how she felt about me driving to which she responded that she was not as comfortable with it as she used to be, however it was she who was now the main driver. He then stated that he did not feel I should be driving any more and he intended to write to the D.V.L.A. in Swansea accordingly. I pointed out to him that my driving licence had recently been re-issued. He in turn pointed out that he had not been consulted on that although I did assure him that I had supplied both his and my G.P.'s names to the D.V.L.A. so I supposed it was their prerogative as to whom they consulted. He then asked for my permission to write to Swansea and I responded that before I agreed I would ask that he support the previous request my G.P. had sent in, at my instigation, for an appointment with either the Ophthalmologist or Neurologist.

These appointments eventually came through but not before the D.V.L.A. had written to me with instructions to return the driving licence they had recently re-issued within three months. The Neurologist confirmed my G.P.'s suspicions.

In addition to the involuntary contractions of my facial muscles, there was also, by now, a tendency to beat my chest with my fists which could only be stopped with great concentrated effort and I was concerned this might be an early indication of either Parkinson's Disease or early symptoms of Alzheimer's. My G.P. however doubted that either was the case but agreed it did require further investigation and the Neurologist was of the same opinion and in turn, following his own examinations, sent me to one of his colleagues, a Psychotherapist at the Radcliffe in Oxford. Over a two hour consultation this doctor put me through a whole series of tests and the only ones that caused him some concern did indeed demonstrate my lack of ability to reverse things through 180° in my mind. I had been aware of this since the first stroke in 1988.

The result of all this research into the problems I had been experiencing was revealed to us some two weeks later by the Consultant Neurologist. I had lost 20% of my brain capacity due to the strokes which he showed us on the pictures from the MRI scan. He observed that I was managing OK with the other 80% and that I had had forty years' worth of damage to the outer sheathing of the nerves from the effects of diabetes. He grinned when I retorted, in my trade terms, "I've been saying for years that I needed a re-wire". He said "yes, but you know as well as I do that it is not possible so just carry on as you always have; it's not stopped you yet and it is certainly not Parkinsons or Alzheimers".

This was obviously a great relief to Joan and myself but a week or so later I was contacted and asked to go back to see the Ophthalmologist who, following some discussion with the Neurologist, had come up with an idea she wished to discuss with me in relation to the muscular contractions I was experiencing around my eyes. She felt this problem may be due to a condition called Blepharospasm which could be overcome by the injection of a toxin that was extracted from snake venom and she gave me a scientific paper to read in order to apprise myself of this condition and its treatment. The treatment was, however, exceedingly expensive and only available in 10cc vials which were only sufficient for two injections, i.e. two separate cases. As I was the only patient available at that time she asked me if I would consider waiting a month or so. I agreed because by now I was convinced that the problem was attributable to my diabetic control.

Following this, Joan and I decided we would spend a couple of weeks walking on Exmoor which we did, averaging ten to fifteen miles each day. Only once was there any problem and that was on the first day after our arrival. An hour or so into our walk my eyes, or rather the muscles round them, contracted and clamped them shut to tightly that Joan had to take me by the hand and lead me across a small pack-horse bridge. A couple approaching from the other side stood and watched us in shock.

A couple of days later I returned the favour. We were approaching a crossing point over the River Exe, at a point indicated on the O.S. map to be a ford, to find that the river was at least waist deep and flowing quite rapidly. Having ascertained there was no alternative crossing point around for some miles I decided to remove my boots and socks and wade across, urging Joan to do likewise. Still maintaining that she could not swim she was obviously very reluctant so I offered to carry her piggy back style across the twenty yards or so to the other side. So that is what I did and on reaching the other side we both sat on the bank with legs outstretched drying in the sun giggling like pre-teen youngsters.

Other than that one incident on the bridge the diabetes gave me no further problems and indeed the regular daily walk cleared the wild fluctuations recorded from the six or seven blood tests I carried out to determine my blood sugar levels. For months past I had been performing these tests on a daily basis and my suspicions were now confirmed. Unless supplemented by physical exercise, insulin had a far greater effect on my nervous system than it did on my blood sugar level. Was this what Robin Lawrence had been referring to in 1960 when he told me that after forty years with the condition things would start to go downhill?

By now the snake toxin I have referred to previously was at last available. However I did inform the Ophthalmologist that the problem had improved with exercise so she decided to inject the dosage into my right eye to see if that would overcome the muscle spasms. I would stress here that the injection was indeed into the eye! Following the injection and with some apprehension at her reaction I told her that her technique and dexterity were terrific and that I had not felt a thing. In the fifteen years or so since I had this procedure unfortunately it did not then or has not since, alleviated this condition which persists intermittently to this day.

Throughout the 1990s my involvement in politics took a back seat after I finished my term as a Councillor in 1992. In early 1993 I became a member of the local Community Health Council and later that year attended the annual conference of health professionals in the sector of diabetes care that was organised by the B.D.A. I was the first lay person, i.e. patient, to do so as a delegate from the Swindon Community Health Council.

On the opening day I caused some concern when I interjected into a rather acrimonious discussion which was taking place between the two disciplines of nursing and doctors. I pointed out that from the point of view of the patient, of which I had, since the age of twelve, now had forty years' experience, we all too frequently found that both disciplines were equally patronising and unprepared to listen and were even less inclined to take account of our observations and experiences. This brought the discussion to an abrupt halt as gasps of surprise echoed around the hall. The Chair subsequently decided to adjourn the meeting for half an hour so that the platform assembly could reflect and consider my observations.

So I made my way to the foyer uncertain of the reception I could expect from others also heading that way. However, to my surprise, I received more praise than admonition with many people remarking that I had made a valid point. One lady with a mid-west American accent enquired if I would be prepared to meet her husband. Intrigued I confirmed that I would be happy to but asked her why. She responded that aside from the diabetes, she felt I had much in common with him and turned to beckon over a man on the staircase who came over and joined us. His name was Jeff and he was the U.K. representative for a Swiss organisation who were introducing an insulin pump which he used himself. He asked me if I would be interested in participating in a trial to which I agreed.

So, three months later, I travelled up to Greenwich where I spent a couple of days with both him and his wife, Bea, at their house. Jeff and I did indeed have a lot in common, both with regard to diabetes, of which I was more senior with regard to duration, and also politics.

Although I took the introduction and instruction course my insistence that I was not prepared to go back onto human insulin resulted in the company to precluding me from the trial. The young tutor was a German lady who was herself a keen walker and swimmer and had been diagnosed with diabetes as a two year old. She was quite taken aback at the company's decision to exclude me from the trials since the thought of someone who had met and been trained by the eminent Dr Lawrence, whom she informed me was revered by the German medical profession, being denied the opportunity staggered her. But despite the efforts of both Jeff and herself the company were not prepared to take what they considered to be too great a risk.

The same decision was confirmed some ten years later following an appointment I had been given at a Bournemouth hospital which was one of the hospitals in the U.K. who were making use of insulin pumps. The Consultant there agreed I was a suitable candidate but only if I was prepared to use human insulin, which I again declined to do.

Some time later I discovered that a fellow member of the Insulin Dependant Diabetes Trust had succeeded in getting onto a pump using animal insulin but by then being well past fifty years on insulin I had lost interest and could not be bothered.

With the disappointment arising from the result of the 1992 General Election my political involvement on any direct basis slipped from my list of primary concerns. This was further enhanced by the death of John Smith, the then Leader of the Labour Party. As a resolute socialist I had no faith whatsoever in the blatant managerial tendencies in respect of capitalism that were so evident in the emerging reformist tendency which subsequently became known as New Labour.

The advent of choice presented to the electorate in 1997 between, what to me was the Tory Party of John Major or the Tory Party of Tony Blair, caused me to fall back on what had always been the approach adopted by the Trade

Unions which was to vote as left as you can. Therefore, on the 1st May 1997, my vote went to Paddy Ashdown's Liberal Party and in two subsequent local elections my vote, on a constituency basis, was cast for either Socialist Unity or the Green Party, since I have no desire to see the continuation of capitalism as an economic system whether allegedly managed in the public interest or otherwise. The whole basis of that system is for individual accumulation of wealth. I believe that man is a social animal and as such must act in the interests of all.

In 1997 Joan did vote for the so-called New Labour, as did millions of others but she very soon realised her mistake and never did so again.

The advent of the millennium did not excite us too much although the early years were marked by one significant event which was the arrival of our granddaughter. When my G.P. had told me to stop working in the early 1990s I had, for a time, occupied myself in the garage making wooden toys for our anticipated grandchildren. I also took up wood turning and marquetry in order to indulge my creative skills and abilities. For a while I used to display and occasionally sell these items at various craft fairs but they were, in the main, distributed throughout the family as presents or placed ornamentally around the home.

My interest in marquetry was initiated when Joan bought me a D.I.Y. kit and I soon become quite adept in this hobby and I could often be found hunting out odd bits of wood veneer and creating my own pictures. Joan, herself, was similarly immersed in her tapestry hobby for which I made her a wood frame to use. The walls of our living and dining rooms are festooned with the results of our efforts.

It was whilst I was working on my lathe in the garage one day in the early 1990s that another new aspects of the long term effects of diabetes again presented itself. I became aware of a feeling of sickness which I initially thought was probably due to dust or vapour in the air as a result of the wood turning I was engaged in. So I put aside the chisel I was using and turned round but the next thing I new I was laid out on the floor underneath the lathe. Out of the corner of my eye I noticed that my glasses were lying on the floor so I reached across my head to retrieve them. As I placed them on my nose I caught sight of blood on my hand which had apparently come from a head wound. Rising to my feet I turned off the lathe and made my way indoors with the intention of using the blood that was oozing from my head to do a BM test. This revealed that I was by no means having a hypo but the blood flow certainly gave Joan a scare.

Our next door neighbour very kindly drove us to the local A&E Department at the hospital where the wound was cleaned and treated. However the medics insisted that I stay in hospital overnight because of a possible concussion. This however proved groundless and the following morning the young doctors who were doing the ward round were all intrigued about my case and asked me numerous questions. Eventually, however, they were summoned away by their senior who was in fact the Consultant I usually saw at the diabetic clinic, whom I have previously referred to. Once these junior doctors were gathered round him raising their observations regarding my case, I caught the words "don't listen to him, he's a nuisance, he will not obey the rules!"

About six months or so after the black out incident I saw the Consultant again at the clinic and he could give no explanation as to the cause of that collapse. However, the scientific papers I had obtained from the B.D.A., the contents of which I had fully absorbed, had not contradicted my own conclusion that insulin had a far greater effect on my autonomic nervous system than my blood sugar. I had diligently recorded and analysed my blood test readings and observations on my daily condition during the course of the previous six months on what are referred to now as spread sheets. However, not being computer literate, I found the damage to the autonomic nerves caused by the then nearly fifty years' duration of living with diabetes in addition to two strokes, caused me more frustration and aggravation than using old fashioned written skills, hence the spreadsheets used my method and work study skills in their presentation.

I then placed this study before the Diabetic Consultant who just swept the papers into the waste bin at the side of his desk dismissing them with a curt comment about the value of old fashioned methods. He again refused to let me have a copy of the letter he had sent to the D.V.L.A. and I had to bite my tongue but resolved, there and then, to do something I had never considered before. If he treated me in this fashion then how the hell would he advise or relate to those newly diagnosed with diabetes? So I wrote a letter of complaint to the Hospital Board. Following a formal investigation the matter was finally resolved via an apology and a mutual acceptance of the fact that between the Consultant and myself our approach to the control of the condition was not compatible, his primary concern being hypo and mine hyperglycemia avoidance. Whilst we both sought to avoid the incidence of long term complications, our approach to doing so differed radically. However he reluctantly admitted that my methods of control had been, and remain, successful in avoiding kidney failure, amputation and blindness. He did think though that only spending about two dozen nights in hospital in the near fifty years I had had the condition did not amount to good control and on that point we agreed to differ.

It was suggested that it might be appropriate for me to transfer my diabetic care to another Consultant and I was give a copy of the letter I had previously sought together with abject apologies for all that had previously transpired. When I later read and absorbed that letter explained the reluctance for me to have a copy and, to a large extent, quite horrified me. It appeared that the Consultant had written to Swansea following a visit to him by both Joan and Dawn who, as he had indicated, was a much respected and knowledgeable Senior Nursing Sister. Both Dawn and Joan had been genuinely concerned that should I be involved in an accident which resulted in others being injured then I would take on the guilt of being responsible for being the cause of serious injury, death or both. Such was my nature that I would probably not be able to live with myself and may take the option that had always been open to me of deliberately taking an insulin overdose.

My initial reaction to this was one of resentment. I could not believe that Joan in particular, of all people, had gone behind my back and been the cause of the loss of my independence which really disappointed me. However, after some harsh words on my part and upon further reflection, I finally realised that both my wife and daughter were right. In many respects these two people probably knew me better than I did myself. Despite the many trials and tribulations my diabetes had thrown my way, my responsibility to my family had always been the reason I had been determined to overcome them. They had both been fearful of my response had I known it was they who had initiated the loss of my driving licence. Their analysis had obviously proven to be correct.

All this had occurred some time before Swansea had actually revoked my licence. Prior to that we had upgraded from the collapsible caravan we had bought to a model where one just elevated the centre section of the roof to give the pair of us the necessary headroom. With Rover discontinuing their Maestro model, which had received the Caravan Towing Vehicle of the Year aware, we took advantage of Derek's entitlement to staff discount as a Rover employee, and bought a two litre diesel model that we got at way below even the discounted end of model price.

So, duly set up with the new unit, we set off for a three week tour of Scotland with myself doing the driving. In that time we covered many areas that were new to both of us in the west and far north putting just over 3,000 miles onto the clock. We had three wonderful weeks in glorious scenery which, as usual, we eagerly explored on foot as well as by car. There were many spots we made a note of to return to on a later visits but, unknown to us at the time, that resolve would never be realised.

The journey home was I think probably undertaken through the worst conditions we had ever encountered since we had joined the A9 near Perth around 9.00 p.m. when we were hit by a gale and driving rain. Driving for the most part through forest it was literally raining fur cones. The noise from this on the van sounded like machine gun fire one hears on either film or T.V. Joan found this experience to be really frightening but I decided to continue driving through the night since the weather showed no signs of easing. In those conditions there was no safe location in which to pull over until we arrived at a motorway service station just north of Birmingham.

The only time I drove after that was at the end of Joan's radiotherapy treatment when I drove the four miles into town and on the return journey was flashed on a number of occasions by several motorists. It was not until I arrived home that I realised why I was being flashed when I found I was having difficulty in judging the distance between the house corner and the wall separating our drive from that of next door. I also realised then why Joan and Dawn had been so concerned. So when I received the letter from Swansea requesting the return of my driving licence three months later I sent it back straight away and resolved to get a bike.

Meanwhile Joan decided to register for a caravan manoeuvring course in order to allow us to continue with our camping holidays. This we were subsequently able to do thanks to her resolute determination despite the fact that arthritis was now starting to cause her increasing trouble. However was equally determined that our walking holidays would continue although we now confined ourselves to the easier heights of Exmoor or the West Sussex woods and downs.

In the mid 1990s Joan quit smoking and, despite all the exercise she got what with housework and our walking weekends, I suppose age was catching up with her and she began to gain weight. This annoyed her intensely as she ate no more than I did yet I did not gain any weight. However I kept assuring her that she still looked great although we were both, by now, as grey as a pair of badgers and I loved her more than ever. At her insistence we confined the celebrations for our Ruby wedding anniversary to just ourselves and the children.

Her weight gain and my diminishing physical capability as a result of the cardiovascular consequences of fifty years' diabetes, was really brought home to the pair of us one morning when she was bringing in the washing from off the washing line and slipped on a patch of moss in the drive and fell heavily onto her knees. Unfortunately I was not at home at the time and the result of her fall was that her left leg was encased in plaster from knee to ankle for a whole month. So I borrowed a wheelchair from Age Concern and would push her around in it to the local parks or shops until the plaster, prettily decorated by our grandchildren, was finally removed. Pushing her on the flat was not too bad but slopes left me really gasping for breath. However I kept assuring her this was due to my heart being under some strain rather than any weight gain on her part. She only just topped eleven stone which was scant comfort to her as she had always maintained a tall size eight. Now, as she entered her sixties, she was disconcerted to discover that her height was making it difficult for her to find a size twelve in clothing, even at "Long Tall Sally" or, to her horror, a size fourteen. Together with Dawn, she would spend hours searching through clothes racks in frustration.

Although we did not know it at the time, fate had even more in store for us. We were both avid readers and regularly visited the library. I would also spend a couple of days each week working on an allotment that was located a couple of miles from our home and had a camping stove there in my shed so that I could make a warming cup of tea or cook some food. I would generally leave for the allotment after breakfast and return in the evening in time for dinner, making my way there and back by bike. Other than the first half mile there or the last half mile on the return journey, the traffic between the estate and village end of this journey was invariably busy and very fast so one had to be very careful and alert.

As I was returning home one evening I turned left into a street leading to the one in which I lived I swung into the middle of the road to avoid a car that was parked on the left hand corner. I checked the length of the street and seeing no further vehicles on the left, swung into the kerb with the intention of cutting across the open grass area leading to my home rather than turn right further along as this route was something of a "rat run". However about fifty metres further on I came to an abrupt halt, sailing forward straight over the handlebars and with a crash found myself bemusedly surrounded by shattered fragments of broken windscreen lying on the boot of a car with my helmet clad head through, of all things, the rear window of a police patrol car! Two men who had been walking on the opposite side of the road had witnessed the incident and immediately called for an ambulance. They came across to extricate me from the patrol car and the ambulance arrived at the same time as the policeman who had been in a nearby house. However I declined to be taken to the A&E Department pointing out that I only lived about two hundred metres away where my dinner would be waiting and also the insulin injection I needed. They reluctantly accepted my decision and after I had signed a medical disclaimer the policeman accompanied me to my home. He told me that his sergeant would call in later in order to take a statement. So later that evening, the statement duly taken, I was assured that in view of my medical condition I would probably hear no more of the incident but I was strongly urged to seriously consider whether I should continue to cycle on the roads, an observation which Joan fully backed up.

Some weeks later Joan accompanied me to the G.P.'s surgery and on the way back I suggested that she drop me off at the allotment and pick me up later that afternoon. I wanted to erect a cane tunnel for our runner beans. This was at around 10.45 a.m.. Placing the individual cans presented me with no problems but reaching up to secure them to each other at the top proved difficult. As it was now approaching lunch time I retreated to the shed to do a blood test and prepare lunch. The blood test revealed that I was neither hypo or hyper, i.e. around seven, so I ate my usual twenty five to thirty grams of carbohydrates and injected thirteen units of long acting insulin.

I had, by experiment over the previous few months, established the cause of the strange effects on my nervous system, upon the suggestion by the Consult-ant that the Protomine Zinc suspension in the bovine may be a factor and as I would not change to synthetic insulin then I should switch to porcine. Now, with the introduction of pens rather than syringes, the opportunity to determine the ratio of short to long term insulin had been taken out of the hands of the patient and vested in the hands of the drug companies. Their pre-mix ratios did not match mine and I had, by experimentation on myself, discovered that the most appropriate time to inject that basal dose was at midday. So, minutes later, I was perched on a camping stool on a patch of concrete adjacent to the shed when I toppled backwards. A short time later I found two men standing over me enquiring if was O.K. I felt a bit strange and disconcerted but managed to do another blood test which revealed that although my blood sugar level was somewhat low I was not technically hypo.

The men asked if they should call an ambulance but I asked if they could first contact Joan, which they did. However as they were becoming increas-ingly concerned at my vagueness and appearance they also rang an ambulance. The two men were not allotment holders so I had to instruct them as to our precise location with directions for the most direct route for the ambulance. They expressed surprise but relayed my suggested route.

Joan arrived just moments before the ambulance and quickly checked to ascertain whether or not I had eaten. She closely examined my eyes and face and satisfied herself that I did not appear to be hypo. When the ambulance arrived the two crew members came forward to where I was sitting on my stool with Joan standing behind me, her hands on my shoulders to keep me steady. The male member of the crew, who knew me, asked if I had eaten anything and wanted to know my most recent BM result. He then turned to his female colleague and asked that she bring the wheeled seat from the ambulance, to which I protested was not necessary. However it was pointed out to me that this was the girl's first call out and was the correct procedure to follow but as he knew me, if I thought I could make it to the ambulance then he would allow me to try but only with their support. So holding my arm and shoulder they raised me to my feet and we started to advance towards the rear of the ambulance. Unfortunately, however, I had only managed about ten yards before I slumped forward to the alarmed cry from the female crew member of "don't do this to me"! Her colleague told her to get the wheeled chair and to fit the ramps to the back of the ambulance where I was quickly taken aboard and with instructions to lie down was then put onto oxygen. Following an examination in A&E I was subsequently told that I had experienced a cardiac arrest twice on that journey to hospital.

Some weeks later I watched fascinated as an angioplasty was performed and, on a monitor, I could see my heart working. To everyone's relief there had been no radical damage but I had to bear in mind the duration of my diabetic condition and perhaps ease off a bit. With that in mind I reluctantly decided to give up cycling, particular in view of my unfortunate incident with the police patrol car. However I was determined to retain my independence and sought to find an alternative, but less strenuous, means of staying mobile. So it was that I acquired a second hand electric powered tricycle from an older man who had previously been a keen motor cyclist but was nervous of using this vehicle on the road as it was only capable of doing fifteen miles per hour. It also offered no protection from either the weather or other road users because it was not equipped to accelerate out of trouble should the need arise. It was, however equipped with lights and indicators and was legally road worthy although restricted to fifteen miles per hour by law. Joan was understandably dubious but understanding my determination to do all I could to maintain my mobility independence, she knew I would do all in my power to do so and despite her misgivings she reluctant accepted this acquisition.

In the meantime her own condition showed no signs of improvement. Her arthritis and IBS (Irritable Bowel Syndrome) meant she had to be treated with a quite powerful analgesic and also, for a time, steroids which obviously had adverse effects on her weight. So we began to lessen our visits to the hills and woods that had previously been our habit as often as we could. Joan rejected the suggestion that perhaps we consider foreign holidays on the grounds that she was quite happy at home provided we were both together. We did have many happy visits to all of our national parks and gained considerable experience of the glories of the U.K. countryside so perhaps we should make more use of our rail passes for day trips.

So this is what we did until well into 2005 when events took a dramatic and completely unexpected turn. Jo developed a quite serious breathing problem which, in her usual way, she dismissed as a heavy cold. However, after a week or so of my continued insistence, she finally made an appointment to see the G.P. with myself accompanying her. The diagnosis she received was that the plural cavity between her lungs and ribs was full of fluid and she needed to attend A&E immediately. So, with Jo driving, we went to the hospital where, following a couple of hours' wait with us both becoming increasingly concerned, four litres of brownish fluid was drained from her plural cavity using one of the largest hypodermic needles I have ever seen. This instantly eased her breathing problem and she was referred to a Pneumococcal Specialist.

A fortnight later we were again in the A&E Department where the same procedure was repeated and a similar amount of fluid extracted. This time, at the next appointment with her Consultant, the suggestion was made that she undergo a minor operation which would enable a camera to be inserted into the plural cavity to examine the area. Additionally, a sealant could also be introduced in the event that any lesion was located. Furthermore, from the last quantity of fluid that had been drained, some unidentified cells had been discovered that needed further examination to determine if they were related to the breast cancer she had had ten years earlier. This procedure would necessitate a four night stay in hospital at Oxford but Joan had received assurances she would be home for Christmas. So she reluctantly agreed and, the procedure completed, we spent a happy Christmas with Dawn and Derek with Katie providing the transport. Joan's breathing was now much easier as a result of the application of the sealant and we had a great time playing board and quiz games with the three grandchildren.

Both of us now felt revitalised and optimistic for the future but this optimism lasted for just three months during which time Jo had returned to her normal happy and efficient self, albeit she was now increasingly concerned about her mother's steady decline. Isobel was now nearing ninety and has started slipping into the initial stages of Alzheimer's. With Jo driving, we would travel down to Pagham once a month which was a ninety mile journey each way. Despite the fact that Isobel was paying Social Services for cleaning help Jo was never happy with the result and would invariably spend the day cleaning whilst I attended the garden which Isobel had already been paying someone to do which gave Joan increasing cause for concern.

However when Joan then received a letter from the hospital with an appointment for her to see the Pneumologist her concerns over Isobel were pushed to the back of our minds. The cells had been identified and whilst sealing the plural cavity had been successful but the Pneumologist told her she needed to see an Oncologist as his specialisation had achieved as much as possible in his field. So Joan was passed onto one of his colleagues who would explain further.

With mounting apprehension we made our way to the Oncology Department where, before anything else was said, we were asked to spend a few minutes with a MacMillan nursing sister. She endeavoured to establish the duration of our relationship, our feelings for each other, medical histories, relatives, etc., and having established the strength of our feelings for each other and other matters considered to be germain to the information we were shortly to be given.

She accompanied us back to the Consultant's office where, once we were all seated, we were told that the rogue cells were not a recurrence of the breast cancer but an indication of lung cancer. Furthermore it would inevitably be terminal. Although we had both been suspicious that lung cancer was a possibility this confirmation came as a hell of a blow, particularly since Jo had shown none of the signs of weight loss and gaunt appearance attributable to the condition that had been apparent when one of my colleagues and his wife before him had also contracted lung cancer. Both had died of the disease some fourteen years earlier.

The Oncologist though did give us some hope in that a course of chemotherapy might arrest the development of the cancer and delay the inevitable. In response to a question from me he said that a determined attitude always helped but chemo could be unpleasant and would only give a delay, not a cure, so the choice was up to Joan. She did not hesitate and responded, nodding in my direction, that she had always told myself and the children that she would live to be a hundred so she had no intention of not trying. With tear rolling down my cheeks we immediately fell into each other's arms and hugged. Joan told me indignantly to stop crying as I would not get rid of her that easily. The Consultant and sister both looked at her in amazement then the sister said "with that attitude Joan, I have the feeling you will be around for a long time yet".

This was in the early summer of 2006. We then had to break the news to Dawn and Derek who were both clearly very upset for, like myself, their worst fears had been confirmed. They now had to deal not only with the emotional stress on themselves but also on their own children. However, all four of us knew that the greatest problem was going to be how to tell Isobel, Joan's mother, so we made arrangements for someone from Social Services to be present when we saw her. In the event, we all came away from that gathering convinced that Isobel had not fully appreciated the gravity of the situation.

Fortunately the chemotherapy did not give Joan too many problems and she managed to hang on to her hair. She had long ceased to be a brunette but still sported a silver grey pageboy cut, much to the envy of many of her younger friends. These women, former D.H.S.S. work colleagues, were all obviously devastated at the news but Joan insisted she wanted to continue with their monthly evenings out for a meal for as long as she could if they were agreeable, which they were. Joan was adamant that these evenings would not be sombre occasions and I subsequently learned that she stamped firmly on any maudling tendencies in the course of conversation.

If my memory serves me correctly, the chemotherapy treatment lasted for approximately ten weeks at the end of which we received the encouraging news that the cancer growth had been arrested. However due to its location, in addition to the problems Joan had experienced with the radiotherapy following the lumpectomy ten years earlier, the possibility of surgery was precluded. We were therefore advised to make the most of the current reprieve.

With that in mind we gave some serious thought to what we would like to do with regard to enjoying some days out. However Jo's primary concern was how and where we would spend what would potentially be our last family Christmas. She had insisted she was going to continue to clean and cook, only trusting me to undertake such tasks as hanging out the washing and occasionally doing some dusting and vacuuming, neither of which I could perform without the odd swear word or exasperated expletive since, Jo being left handed, the vacuum hose would invariably be coiled in the opposite direction to what I wanted as I was right handed.

She also endeavoured to continue to drive so once again I borrowed a wheel chair for her so that I could push her round the supermarket. At that stage there were very few things she would not attempt to do being quite indignant on occasions when I either tried to assist or perform the task for her.

The question of Christmas was resolved by everyone congregating at Dawn's who thoughtfully sought her mother's advice on preparing dinner for the nine of us who had gathered there. Isobel had been transported from Bognor to Dawn's home in Warwickshire for what we all expected to be Joan's last Christmas which she wanted to spend with all those she loved, i.e. her mother, husband, children and grandchildren.

Needless to say that festive season was extremely emotional and incredibly hard for all of us but we made the most of it and tried our utmost to remain positive. Joan, Dawn, Derek and myself were only too well aware that this might well be our last Christmas together and we really had to fight to stay dry eyed. However the quiz games we played in the evenings provided some light relief and joy as our grandchildren vied with each other to partner their nanny which helped to lift our spirits.

Following Christmas and as the weather improved our thoughts turned to possible coach trips we could enjoy. There were two that particularly appealed to us the first of which was a trip to the Chelsea flower show which we had thoroughly enjoyed twenty years previously on our first and only trip there. The second was a combination trip to the London Eye and a boat ride from Westminster to Greenwhich. This latter would allow us to see how much the waterfront had changed since we left London and also to possibly repeat some of our regular evening strolls from our courting days now nearly fifty years previously.

We subsequently decided that the Chelsea trip would not be possible since we felt the crowds would present a problem so as an alternative we decided to visit Kew Gardens, a venue we had never previously gotten round to visiting. This proved to be something of an adventure in itself because the coach driver took a route that came as a complete surprise to me and my continuous puzzling over the route and second guessing where we were going to end up eventually got on Jo's nerves. However when we finally reached our destination the gardens themselves proved to be utterly delightful. Jo had reluctantly agreed with my suggestion that I borrow a wheelchair from the Kew Red Cross Depot which would enable us to see as much as possible. We had taken along a picnic lunch and the weather was good so we enjoyed everything we were able to see. I must admit though I was really thrown by the quality of the vegetable patch which made my own feeble efforts pale in comparison. As always, Jo attempted to raise my spirits by pointing out that the land at Kew did not consist of heavy clay!

At about 3.30 p.m., after visiting the many glasshouses and marquees housing the vast collections of a variety of different plants, we made our way back to the entrance where we could get a cup of tea and meet up with the coach which was due to leave at 4.15.p.m. As we approached the entrance the Red Cross office, from which I had borrowed the wheelchair, came into view. It being a hot day we both wanted a drink of water, the more so since Joan needed to take some pills which she could never manage to do without a drink. As I pushed her towards the office she became increasingly alarmed at our unsteady progress and when we eventually got there she asked the woman inside to provide me with some sugar as a matter of urgency. As per usual she had instantly recognised the signs that I was hypo but, also as usual, I was determined, come hell or high water, to achieve my objective which this time was to get my beloved wife to where she could get a cool drink. The alarmed woman at the Red Cross office met both our needs and listened somewhat perplexed as Joan answered her questions and explained our circumstances healthwise. So with her very best wishes and professed admiration to our approach to our situation ringing in our ears we eventually left the office and made our way, hand in hand, back to the coach.

A couple of hours later the driver dropped us off close enough to home to allow us to walk the half mile there. It had been a great day out and that evening we discussed the day's events and made plans for our second planned coach outing some ten days hence.

This second trip would see us take a launch from Westminster pier down to the Millenium Dome and back following which we would take a flight on the London Eye. Joan, although sceptical of this latter arrangement, was prepared to give it a try.

Once again the weather was kind to us and on this occasion we had decided to rationalise to the extreme what we would need to carry with us so our baggage this time consisted solely of glucose tablets and a small bottle of water. We decided would dine and get a drink at a convenient pub or restaurant rather than take our own lunch thereby breaking the habit of a lifetime dictated by my diabetes. However in the circumstances and in view of Joan's situation that was the least of my concerns although Jo took some convincing as to its practicality.

The coach dropped us off on the embankment, a matter of yards from Westminster pier, and our attention was immediately drawn to two features that were new to us, neither of which had been there fifty years earlier when, in our courting days, we took our regular late night walks making our way back to Vauxhall following an evening out. The first of these was the commando memorial. Whilst not making it into the unit, Joan's father, Albert, had undergone his infantry training at their school in the Scottish highlands. The second was the Battle of Britain memorial plaque, the relief carving of which impressed us both.

We eventually managed to tear ourselves away and descend to the pier where we boarded and managed to find a couple of vacated seats at the front of the launch. However we very soon realised why these seats had been vacated as there was quite a chill breeze blowing upstream from the estuary way off to the east. Once we had passed the all too familiar sights of County Hall and the Festival Hall on the south bank we began to realise just how much the waterfront had changed as we neared Blackfriar's Bridge.

This continued to be the case until we approached Tower Bridge when, in the main, the perceived changes switched from the south to the north bank. Then, we both gasped in surprise as Tower Bridge started to open and we gazed in amazement as the reason for this revealed a Mississippi paddle steamer progressing mid stream. As both the left and right sides of the bridge were slowly raised we laughed in delight and, for a moment, thought how our grandchildren would love to be taken for a trip on that but then reflected it was an unlikely desire. At that point a photographer approached us and Joan asked him to take our picture. That picture, taken on that launch in the middle of the Thames, was to give us both a great deal of pleasure over the next few months. It really expressed our deep love for each other which now, in our sixties, was every bit as intense as when I had similarly asked a stranger to take our picture in our teens when we had been on the embankment opposite Lambeth Palace.

When we arrived back at Westminster we disembarked and made our way to what I believe is known as St Steven's Tavern, for lunch and a drink. On entering I was surprised to see a couple of faces I recognised from the rate capping discussions twenty years earlier. They likewise also reciprocated this recognition but other than exchanging greetings and good wishes I made it clear it would be inappropriate to continue such discussions, given the circumstances, so I placed our orders and returned to sit at a table Joan had found.

With lunch over we made our way across Westminster Bridge to the London Eye where we joined the queue. It now being quite warm we decided to have an ice cream after which we stood puzzling over the strange garb of a couple of girls nearby and a man looking for all the world like ghosts! I could only surmise that we had unwittingly wandered onto a film set but at my suggestion the man indignantly proclaimed they were performing artists, much to Joan's amusement. Thus corrected and diplomatically reprimanded I took Joan's hand and led her onto the ramp leading up to the loading platform for the capsules on the London Eye. I assured her that the sensation would be a lot less disconcerting than using a lift, which she hated and would always avoid if at all possible. So she agreed to try and, apart from the brief change in direction between the twelve and one o'clock rotation, at the end of the flight she admitted that the experience had not been as bad as she had initially feared. However once was enough and, "no", she did not want to go around again later!

For both of us the flight on the Eye had been very pleasant as we had been able to identify familiar landmarks including the block of flats where Joan had grown up, the senior school she had attended, the approximate location of the flat where we had spent the first nine months of our married life, the church we were married in and the pub at the Oval where we had held our reception. Sadly however I could see no trace of my home in Peckham or indeed the surrounding streets since the whole area had given way to the North Peckham Estate.

After we left the Eye we decided to walk along the south bank although as we passed Waterloo it was becoming apparent that neither of us was finding it easy. I was now using a walking stick and needed to pause every hundred yards or so. Whilst Joan refused to use a stick she welcomed these pauses, not only to gather breath and strength herself but also to ease the pressure on her hips. We did however manage to make it as far as Blackfriars but then, to the disappointment of us both, used as we were to our past ten or twelve mile treks across fells or moors three years earlier, we agreed that we would have to turn back. To try to proceed any further would inevitably cause one or both of us a serious problem as neither of us was capable any longer of physically assisting each other for more than a few yards.

This indeed subsequently proved to be the case. As we approached the green area to the side of County Hall, alongside which, at its southern end, stood a line of parked coaches, Joan came to a sudden stop unable to go any further. At the end of the path, around the edge of the green area, I noticed a number of benches and at my insistence, for she was very reluctant, I urged my wife to put her right arm around my neck and lean against me. Placing my left arm under her left armpit to support her we eventually made it to the bench nearest to the line of coaches. A couple that were sitting there looked up in alarm as we approached and shuffled along to make room for us. Once Joan was seated and I established that a nice cup of tea would be welcome I made my way to a nearby kiosk. Fortunately this beverage was served in beakers with a snap-tight lid so by balancing them on a reasonably stiff plate in place of a tray, although with some difficulty, I made my way back to her.

To an extent this welcome cup of tea and the short rest refreshed her and having established that the coach on the near end of the line was the one we wanted, with myself supporting Joan in the manor adopted to reach the bench, we covered the four or five hundred yards to board it. Having discovered the reason for our difficult approach, when we arrived back in Swindon, the kindly driver made a point of dropping us off outside our home. Although we had had a really nice day, it had been brought home to us that Joan's condition was deteriorating.

That night, as had usually been the case, she really struggled to climb the stairs to bed and I had to support her by following behind to ensure she did not fall. She was now habitually using the downstairs toilet, the seat of which I had endeavoured to raise but whilst this was of some help she was losing the strength to raise herself up from it and frequently needed my assistance. This concerned her for not only did she find it humiliating because she was not losing weight, she feared my lifting her would place too much strain on my back or heart. Despite my protests to the contrary she was more concerned at my situation than her own. So it was, after some reluctance on Joan's part, that we agreed to contact the Oncologist to establish what was happening. A scan subsequently revealed that the cancer had started to grow again and he was dubious that a second course of chemotherapy would prove as successful as the first. Additionally, in Joan's weakened state, it would be far more unpleasant for her so after leaving us alone to discuss matters Joan emphasised that she wanted to die at home. She now felt that everything possible had been done medically and we now had to face up to the reality of the situation together. Whilst I accepted Joan's wishes I in my turn emphasised to her that we must accept what material assistance Social Services or the medical profession could offer.

Thus it came about that a hospital bed was delivered to the house and liquid morphine prescribed. With her usual reluctance to take medication it was only with a great deal of persuasion from both myself and the community matron, who came every three days, that she finally agreed to take the medication. She argued that all it did was make her tired and she felt tired enough already.

It was on one of her visits one morning that the matron, intrigued but impressed by my efforts to modify the toilet seat for Joan, remarked that what was really needed was a frame to place over the toilet which incorporated a raised seat and side arms. So following a telephone call to the N.H.S. depot to establish that one was available, she was informed that it would have to be collected. Having told her that I could not use the car parked on the drive the matron was taken aback when I announced I would collect it using my trike or a bus and she suggested that a taxi was the obvious solution. Since I resolutely rejected that suggestion she sought to persuade me to change my mind. Jo intervened with "don't waste your breath, I've been trying for nearly forty seven years but if he says he will do it then he will"!

However the problem was overcome when Derek, who was working day shift, eventually drove me to the depot in his lunch break. Whilst we were there we also collected a swivel shower seat to allow Joan to use our shower that was mounted over the end wall of the bath. As it transpired, however, she was only able to do this on a few occasions.

Joan's main concern now became saying goodbye to her mother which was made doubly difficult by the emotional shock it would cause and the fact that Isobel would then be left alone in her bungalow. To try to overcome this we contacted the lady at West Sussex Social Services whom Joan had first contacted in relation to her mother, to ask that she be in attendance when we gave her mother the bad news. This she agreed to do so a few days later Derek drove his mother and I down to Pagham for, we anticipated, this final goodbye since it was now clear that Joan was getting weaker. She was, however, determined to say goodbye to her mother on her own terms whilst she was still capable of doing so. She also wanted to assure herself that her mother's future care was taken care of which was being arranged between West Sussex and Warwickshire Social Services since Dawn would now be taking on the responsibility for her grandmother as Joan would soon be unable to continue in that capacity.

In her last few weeks, as always, Joan was more concerned about her loved ones than herself. Indeed, a couple of nights later, lying on the hospital bed in our living room, she grasped my hand from where I was trying to sleep on the settee beside her. I was up immediately anxiously trying to establish what was wrong, checking her pulse and brow and raising the upper end of the bed a little. She said "Tony, I want you to promise me you will keep going when I am gone." I protested that I would have no desire to do so without her but she in turn responded with "I know love, I have been there a number of times with you over the last forty six years but you have always told me that it was your love for me and the children that pulled you through. I know you have always had it in your power to secure your exit. What I need you to promise is that you won't. I cannot keep going much longer and I cannot die happy love until I have your promise. Neither the children or grandchildren should have to face losing us both close after each other".

The effects of over fifty years with diabetes and its subsequent effects on my automonic nervous system, particularly my eyelids and facial muscles, were now dire, being at its worst following my morning injection. The resultant feelings of dejection and despair that would overwhelm me between 8.00 a.m. and 10.00 a.m. when I would habitually carry a cup of tea into Joan were only lifted from me by our loving interaction. I would nudge her shoulder to wake her and she would invariably twist her head and shoot me a slightly mocking yet grateful grin. However I was none too sure that, overwhelmed with grief as I knew I would be when the inevitable happened, I would be able to keep such a promise she had asked me to make. I put these doubts to Joan and through her tears she said "I know it will be hard love but I need you to promise that if it should happen that you follow soon after me then it will not be deliberate. Promise me that". Hearing her say those words made me realise that Joan had understood what a difficult decision she was asking of me and I also realised why she was pushing me. From the moment I had first held Joan in my arms, then Dawn and two years later Derek, I knew I had a reason to determinedly overcome all the problems life and diabetes had thrown our way. In building, providing and defending all the love and devotion Joan had given to us she knew she was inevitably going to lose the ability to do so soon but her sole concern now was to do all in her power to ensure I continued on. In a blinding flash I knew why she was pushing so hard to extract that promise from me. She knew, probably better than I knew myself, that I would never break a promise I had made to her.

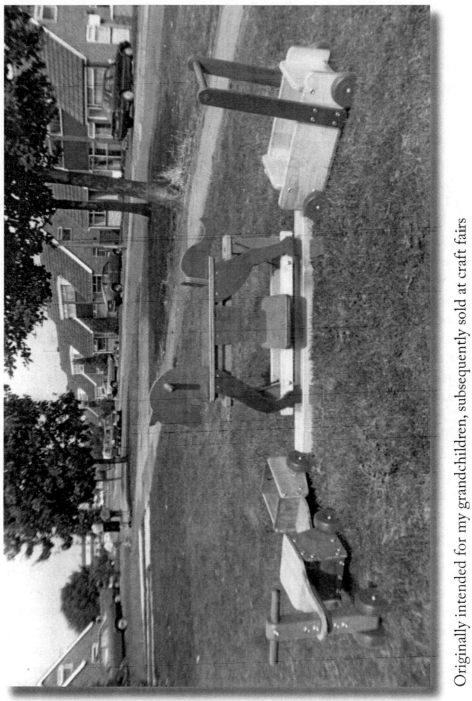

Originally intended for my grandchildren, subsequently sold at craft fairs

Loss of Joan

Over the course of that last week she had been very reluctant to eat. Even meals I had liquidised through the blender proved difficult for her as she was now suffering with constipation. When two attempts with an enema administered by the District Nurses proved unsuccessful they informed me they could not proceed any further without a doctor in attendance. Therefore, in some trepidation and great concern, I contacted our G.P.'s surgery first seeking then demanding a doctor's visit. The doctor duly arrived some minutes later, listened to the nurses' report then proceeded to examine Joan. Turning to me he then, to my disappointment, informed me that she was now too ill to be cared for at home and given my condition, i.e. the diabetes, he would have to send her to hospital. I protested and asked if she could be sent to the hospice instead which he agreed would be more appropriate. Unfortunately however he had already established that at that time there were no beds available but Joan was top of the list should one become available. So an ambulance was summoned and such was my anxiety in accompanying her that I left the house without my insulin.

Upon arrival at the hospital Joan was placed in the Acute Admission Unit and the MacMillan Sister, Jane, from the Oncology Department was summoned. She informed us that Joan's grossly bloated stomach was due to trapped gas which her stomach acids continued to produce despite the fact that she had not eaten anything for two days. She told Joan to forget her ladylike behaviour and try to pass wind! In order to allow her to do so Jane would try to get her moved to a single patient room which would also facilitate the family to visit. She further urged Joan to take the morphine she had been given which would make it a bit easier for her. As she had bravely faced the outcome of her situation and its inevitability, the morphine would also enable her to say goodbye in comfort. So, after being settled into a single bed room, Joan then turned to me and asked if I had bought my injection kit with me. When I replied that I did not her concern immediately switched from herself to me. Assuring me she had no intention of going yet she ordered me to go home and get it with the instruction to tell the children and return in the morning.

So I returned home and informed both Dawn and Derek that their mother was now in hospital. During that night I contacted the hospital on numerous occasions to check on Joan's condition, returning to her there the next morning. To my joy I found she was reasonably bright and determined to remain that way since both Dawn and Derek had telephoned to let her know they would be bringing in the grandchildren to see her. They subsequently arrived striving hard to remain cheerful and positive but I don't think any of them fully realised just how ill Joan was. She, in her own right, was determined to preserve the myth that she would soon be home and accepted a number of jelly babies the girls offered to her. Her message to Alex, Gemma and Katie was to try their best at school and be good. Listening to this and observing Joan's positive approach, I followed the nurse who had been attending her out of the room. When I asked her what the situation was she responded that she thought Joan's time was near and the doctors were seeking to move her out of A.A.U. to either a ward or a hospice.

I returned to the room with tears streaming down my cheeks and sat down taking Joan's hand in mine. The others looked at me in some concern but Joan said as indignantly as she could "What are you crying for, I'm not gone yet?" Following a brief word with Derek, Dawn then decided to check with the doctor and sister and, with her own extensive experience, told them it was not yet appropriate to use a morphine pump. After the emotion of the last few hours, Joan indicated that she was tired and wanted to sleep. Squeezing my hand she said "I'll see you in the morning love, it's not time yet".

The following morning I found Joan in a four bed ward, only three of which were occupied. She was awake and managed a smile when she saw me and indicated she wanted to be raised up. She put her arms round my neck as I slipped my arm behind her shoulders and as I straightened up the nurse slipped a couple of pillows behind her. Jo released her arms from around my neck, grasped and squeezed my left hand and as I leaned forward to kiss her she gasped in my ear "Tony, keep your promise". These were to be the last words my darling wife was to say to me for at that moment a doctor appeared and stepping forward asked Joan if he could take her husband away for just a moment to have a word with me to which she nodded her head. I followed the doctor to an office where he told me that Joan now had pneumonia in both lungs. As he said this the telephone rang and after a conversation lasting about four minutes he replaced the receiver and told me that had been the hospice. However he told me that neither he nor his colleague at the hospice felt that Joan would be able to survive the journey there which would only cause her unnecessary suffering with no possible advantage. He then asked for my permission to use the morphine pump and said it would be set at its lowest setting when I responded that our children were on their way.

I returned to Joan's side and took her hand which gripped and squeezed mine in response. Her face tightened with the effort as we reaffirmed with each other what a great life we had shared over the fifty years since we had first met and how much we loved each other. My sister, Colleen, then arrived together with our niece and two nephews, having driven down from London. They stayed for half an hour or so, each exchanging a few words with Joan until with a nod from their mother tactfully withdrew. I glanced at Colleen as I became aware that Joan's grip on my hand was lessening and as I squeezed her hand and raised my head our eyes met and held briefly as she slipped away and I lost the love of my life.

I began sobbing my heart out as both Dawn and Derek arrived ten minutes later, having been caught in traffic. They both let out a grief stricken howl and bent down to kiss their mother goodbye for the last time stroking her hair as they did so. Dawn bravely took command of the situation and ushered myself and her brother to the foot of the bed where all three of us stood with our arms wrapped around each other the tears rolling down our cheeks, our bodies racked with grief. Knowing what was inevitably going to happen did not make our loss any easier to bear.

However I realised there was one last thing that Joan had wanted me to do for her so disentangling myself from my son and daughter I made my way to the head of the bed and gazing for the last time into my wife's beautiful hazel eyes I lifted my hand and closed her eyelids. With this final loving duty performed and with my tears falling onto her face, in accord with her wishes I raised her left hand to my mouth and wetting her finger withdrew her engage-ment, eternity and wedding rings. As per Joan's wishes, I gave her engagement ring to Dawn and the wedding ring to Derek.

On Joan's right hand she wore the last of the three wedding rings we had purchased as a result of her fingers swelling since I had placed the original one on her finger forty seven years previously. I had given her the eternity ring on our tenth wedding anniversary and I asked Dawn to place this, together with the third wedding ring, onto the chain around my neck which held my identity disc. They will remain there, close to my heart, for ever more.

July has always been an auspicious month that not one of us was over fond of. This was even more true now as not only had I lost my father on the 4th July, twelve years earlier, but now on the 3rd July, 2007, I had also lost my wife as well. I now had to face my sixty ninth birthday on the 9th July alone and it would by no means be a happy one.

The immediate concern now was to find a humanist officiant for whilst I had every intention of writing Joan's eulogy myself, as indeed I had for both my parents, there was no way I would be able to read it as I knew my grief would be too much and I would be in far too an emotional state crying my eyes out. However we were fortunate enough to find a very nice lady whom we knew would perform this task with respect and sympathetic understanding.

On the occasion of Joan's funeral, the details of which we had both discussed sometime previous, her only stipulation had been that she be cremated and the 23rd Psalm be played to the music of Crimond as it had at our wedding. She had also wanted the entrance of her coffin to be made to "Didn't it Rain?" sung by Mahalia Jackson and her exit to "Every time we say goodbye" by Ella Fitzgerald. She had also stipulated that the reading be Shakespeare's 116 Sonnet which summed up our feelings for each other.

With Dawn and Derek supporting each other they managed to deliver their own eulogies to their mother but I had to rely on the officiant to read what I had written whilst I sat shaking with my sobs of grief. When we went outside afterwards Joan's friends and colleagues all rallied round with expressions of sympathy and deep regret at the loss of their friend and mentor. Joan had been some twenty years older than most of them and each one had very much valued her advice and knowledge when they had confronted her with their problems.

However I was really brought up short when Ginge, a friend I had not seen for some years, placed an arm round my shoulders and made me realise that our children, grandchildren and Joan's mother, Isobel, were also in desperate need of comforting. He pointed out that in my grief I had not realised how lucky I was to have had a love affair that had lasted for fifty years. Very few people experienced that happiness or had that wealth of memories. For a moment I stood their shocked before accepting the truth of his words whereby I then gave my full attention to our offspring. That evening the whole family gathered on the drive, all seventeen of us, as we circulated photographs we had taken over the past fifty years, reminiscing about all those wonderful memories.

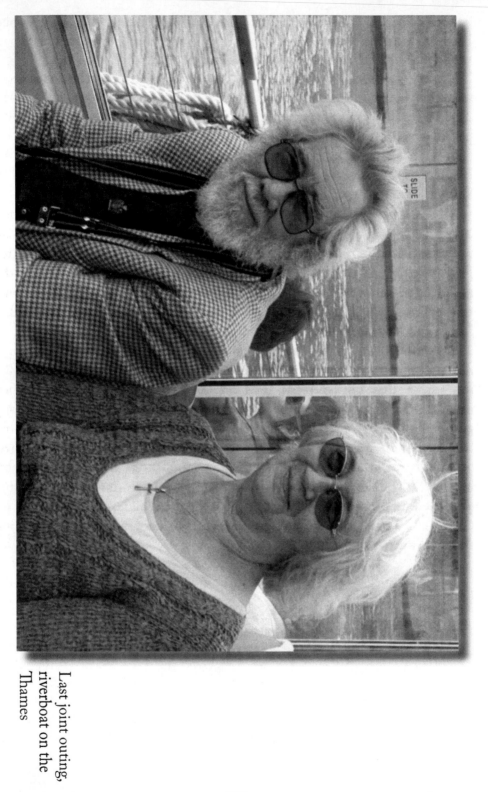

Last joint outing, riverboat on the Thames

Attempting to Keep my Promise

The question was finally raised about I would now manage on my own and whether I should consider moving. However I made it clear that I had no intention of breaking the promise I had made to Joan who, during her last few weeks, had urged me not to make any hasty decisions with regard to moving. She knew I would be bored out of my mind if I did not have the opportunity of losing myself in some project or other in either the garage or the garden. There was one obvious problem however that did need to be addressed and that was what would happen in the event I had a hypo whilst I was asleep. In the forty six years Joan and I had shared a bed this had happened numerous times but the times that Joan had needed to seek medical assistance had been very few and far between. I now had to explore possible ways to overcome this potential problem.

I was aware of developments in electronic monitoring and alarm systems. Some fifteen years earlier I had initiated the Home Line alarm system in the borough when I was Council Leader. As a District Council this was beyond our remit but despite that and also rate capping, this did not prevent us from instituting what was a County Council responsibility. This was only one of the many responsibilities that the Tory controlled Wiltshire County Council failed to provide in the Swindon area. However Swindon was now a Unitary Authority with statutory responsibility for Social Services so I contacted that department to ascertain what equipment may be available to help overcome the potential problem of nocturnal hyperglycemia.

Following some discussions between myself and an officer from that department, together with a second officer who, at my request, brought along a catalogue of the alarm equipment available, we agreed on two items that could provide a warning that was linked to a central location in the event of me experiencing a hypo. This would be sent via a radio link I could wear that would send a signal in the event of me falling. They could also provide an enuresis detector which is placed under the sheet on my bed and detects excessive sweating associated with nocturnal hypos. If I did not react to an incoming telephone call from the central location an ambulance would immediately be summoned. This whole procedure only needed a telephone line with the only external element being the need to install a key safe and security number to allow a paramedic to gain access to the house in the event that I may be unconscious.

So it was that just a month after Joan's death this equipment came into its own. I was outside working in the garden planting broad bean seeds down the side of the greenhouse. I was methodically working across the outside rear of the greenhouse, the earth being quite damp, and as I reached the rear left hand corner I placed my left hand on the corner for support. It was close to lunch time so I knew I would soon need to stop to have something to eat. However at that point I began to lose control of my legs and as my right foot flexed forward onto the damp ground it slipped away from me thus throwing the weight of my body onto my outstretched left arm. I span round on that arm back into the rear wall of the greenhouse smashing the glass from top to bottom. I slid to the ground writhing around in shards of broken glass struggling to undo the button of my shirt pocket to get to my glucose tablets. The fall detector went off and within ten minutes two paramedics were hauling me to me feet. I was taken to A&E where it became apparent that a shard of glass was embedded deep in my left buttock. This was going to need surgical attention as the A&E doctors were unable to extract it. In order to achieve this the surgeon suggested I be put on an insulin drip which would have to be synthetic as opposed to animal insulin. I refused and argued it should be done without anaesthetic since the damage to my auto-monic nervous system had resulted in a greatly reduced sensitivity to pain. At the end of extensive discussions in this regard it was decided that I should have an epidural injection to the base of my spine so throughout the procedure I remained conscious.

The young daughter of the Anaesthetist had recently been diagnosed with Type One diabetes and I was able to pass on to her what she assured me had been very useful advice that had the added value of allowing me to survive for fifty years with the condition as proof of its validity.

A shard of glass some thirty millimetres long and ten millimetres wide at its base was removed from my buttock and the resulting wound was packed and stitched. Ten days later I returned to hospital for the injury to be examined and the surgeon was amazed that the wound was clean and had completely healed. Once again I was complimented on my management of the condition.

Some six months later, however, I received something of a shock when I went into our downstairs utility room to use the toilet and felt very unsteady. So I deliberately shrank to the floor and crawled into the living room where I knew there was a Mars Bar in a low cupboard accessible from the floor. I managed to locate it and eat half, by now sweating profusely. However this did not appear to be having any effect but try as I might I just could not raise myself to my feet. As my condition was not improving I started to become concerned. Remembering my promise to Joan that I would keep going I crawled into the dining room and hit the panic button. As a voice came through I tried to explain that I was now in a situation that I could not manage and asked for an ambulance to be summoned. I then crawled back into the laundry room, reached up and opened the rear door just as a paramedic accessed the key safe. He entered and carried out a blood test and smeared my gums with a hypostop. He then handed me an oxygen mask as his colleague brought in a wheelchair. Together they helped me to remove the sweat soaked cardigan I was trying to take off and took me out to the ambulance. It was now an hour since I had eaten dinner.

At the hospital, following an initial ECG, I was put onto a heart monitor for twenty four hours. In my confused, or preoccupied, state the previous evening I had neglected to ask the paramedics to fetch my insulin from the fridge. I declined the synthetic insulin from the hospital's stock, skipped both breakfast and lunch, so my body was running on the long acting insulin I had injected some twenty two hours previously. As this was available I injected my usual dose at midday. My blood sugar reading was eleven as a result of the effects of the half Mars Bar and hypostop administered seventeen hours earlier.

In the late afternoon it became clear from the results of the blood tests that were taken at intervals since my admission, that I had not had a heart attack. However the doctors wanted me to stay in hospital until I had been seen by a Cardiologist which unfortunately could not be for at least another twenty four hours at the earliest. By now porcine insulin was available but the only food available was a sandwich so, following some discussions with the doctors, I announced it was my intention to see the Cardiologist as an outpatient and would be discharging myself, which was strictly against medical advice. Knowing I had a cooked meal in the freezer at home I ate no food until I after I had returned home and injected my normal insulin dose.

So, it being November, I borrowed a blanket to wrap around my shoulders and managed to catch a bus home, also getting a telling off from the driver for discharging myself. At last I had a decent hot dinner. Since losing Joan I had got into the habit of cooking casseroles large enough to provide me with three meals, one of which I would eat straight away and the other two I would put into the freezer.

Two weeks later I saw the Cardiologist who informed me there was no evidence of further damage to my heart following the recent incident but he also told me that heavy sweating was also associated with heart attacks as well as hypoglycemia. I responded with "C'est la vie" (that's life) at which he grinned and agreed that yes it did indeed make things awkward for me but that I seemed to be managing it well and to keep it up.

After I had discharged myself from hospital I had been amazed when I got home to find that my cardigan was still wringing wet hanging over the back of the toilet where I had discarded it nearly thirty hours previously despite the central heating being left on. I was however relieved to discover my glasses lying undamaged on the floor where they had been dislodged from my sweat soaked face as I had crawled round the floor.

The Cardiologist and the Diabetic Consultant, whose clinic I attended, had discussed my recent incident and were both of the opinion that the cause was probably an anti-rhythm of the heart that had occurred as a result of a hypo coupled with the damage to my autonomic nervous system following nearly sixty years with diabetes. I had been fortunate at the start of my diabetes to have come under the auspices of the great Doctor Lawrence and now, some sixty years later, was still fortunate in seeing another Diabetic Consultant who was always open to discussion and prepared to listen. His name was Doctor Sahid Ahmed who has often told me that I have always been prepared to carry out experiments on myself in relation to treatments, etc., that he would have suggested to me before he was given the opportunity to do so. The lessons that had been learned as a result had indeed served us both. For my part I have a great deal off respect for this man which is also shared by many others under his care.

In the sixty years I have had this condition the number of times I have required urgent medical assistance and the number of nights I have had to spend in hospital as a result amount to no more than can be counted on the digits of both hands and feet. In the main this achievement is due to three factors.

Firstly, as a twelve year old, I received a sound education on managing and living with diabetes which I have adhered to and built upon from experience.

Secondly, as a nineteen year old, I met a wonderful girl who, after a three year courtship, became my wife. It was her love and belief in me that fuelled my determination that the condition would not beat me.

Finally, I believe it has been my sheer pig headedness not to be beaten, a trait I believe I must have inherited from my father.

Give or take three units, I am still injecting the same forty units of insulin per day that I was prescribed sixty years ago and eating two thirds of the daily carbohydrate requirement I consumed at the start and throughout my working life.

Now, as a seventy two year old, despite the fact that, for a variety of reasons, my mobility ability precludes me from getting the same degree of exercise, the lesson from the account of my life is clear:-

1. Maintain strict control of your carbohydrate intake.
2. Learn to balance insulin and exercise.
3. Do not let it beat you.

If you follow this doctrine you can manage it and have a great, happy and fulfilling life, despite the diabetes.

How I learned to live with diabetes

Tony tells of the choice he was given as a boy

TONY Huzzey was given a stark choice at the age of 12 - either accept the fact that he would have to inject himself four times a day or die.

Electrician Mr Huzzey, who is now 60 and a former leader of Thamesdown Borough Council, recalls the first time he fell ill with what was to be diagnosed as type one diabetes.

Type one diabetes tends to begin in childhood, while type two diabetes tends to begin in adulthood.

Mr Huzzey said: "I had become seriously ill and my GP was baffled because he had limited experience of dealing with diabetes.

"I was admitted to Kings College Hospital, London, where I was lucky to be seen by a doctor who recognised that I had diabetes, because he had the same condition himself.

"I was told that I had been about 36 hours from death.

"When I was sufficiently recovered, I was told quite bluntly that I had to accept the fact that I would have to live with diabetes, which would involve regulating my diet and injecting insulin.

"The alternative was that I would die. It was quite a lot to take on board at the age of 12, but as the eldest child of three I knew I had to set an example and do as I was told."

Mr Huzzey, of Hawkswood, Covingham, remembers being given a set of needles to inject himself with.

"On my first occasion, I was given a piece of rubber tube to practise on for two hours and then it was up to me to inject myself.

"There was no question about my parents having to do it for me. I was encouraged to take responsibility for my own condition. My doctor laid down the ground rules which I have followed to this day."

Mr Huzzey, who has two children and three grandchildren, attributes his having lived in relatively good health for 48 years to the advice he was given as a boy.

He said: "I very quickly had to learn the amount of carbohydrate that I could eat, and I would advise my mother. It was all a bit of a mystery to her."

Mr Huzzey's self-administered treatment has become second nature. Each morning before breakfast he tests his blood sugar level, using a small needle to break the skin and a measuring device.

He then injects a long-lasting and short acting dose of insulin. Further injections throughout the day include a further dose before lunch and one before bed.

He said: "I take my own health seriously and ensure that I maintain my blood sugar level very carefully. People with type two diabetes tend to have problems sometimes, because they are not as disciplined about their care.

"The key is about taking responsibility."

USEFUL NUMBERS:
Diabetes UK (0207) 4241000
Diabetes Care Line (0207) 7424 1030
NHS Direct (0845) 4647

INTERNET LINKS
www.diabetes.org.uk
www.nhsdirect.nhs.uk

■ My doctor laid down the ground rules which I follow to this day . . . Tony Huzzey   Picture: MATTHEW SWINGLER Ref: 25080-1

Millions are undiagnosed

AS part of Diabetes Week - June 7 to 13 - charity Diabetes UK is highlighting the fact that there are more than a million undiagnosed people with the condition.

If you have the following symptoms, which are a possible indicator of diabetes, you should see your GP: lethargy, constant thirst, frequent need to urinate, weight loss, blurred vision, numb fingers or toes, repeated fungal infections.

Diabetes occurs when the body fails to produce enough of the hormone insulin to remove glucose from the blood.

Because there is not enough insulin, glucose remains in the bloodstream, causing raised blood sugar levels.

There are two types of diabetes.

Type one diabetes usually develops in childhood when the body fails to produce insulin. Treatment is in the form of injections of insulin and careful regulation of the diet.

Type two diabetes develops later in life and occurs when cells in the body become resistant to insulin, even though the hormone is being produced. Treatment is by diet regulation, medication - and in the most extreme cases insulin injections.

The number of people suffering from this type of diabetes is soaring in developed countries.

The rise is thought to be caused by increasing levels of obesity, which has been linked to the condition.

FACT FILE

■ More than three in every 100 people in the UK have been diagnosed with diabetes, about 1.4 million people. A further million people have the condition without realising it.

■ Diabetes cannot be cured, but it can be controlled.

■ Diabetes is not caused by eating too many sugary foods.

■ Diabetes is not infectious.

■ People with diabetes do not necessarily go blind in their old age, contrary to what many people believe. The condition can eventually cause retinopathy – impaired vision due to damaged blood vessels in the retinas - which can be treated with laser therapy.

Article in local paper in 2003, prompted by request from Diabetes UK to do an interview

••• 258 •••

Concluding Thoughts

Looking back over the past sixty years I suppose I would have to admit that my greatest disappointment is the failure of those of us on the left to convince the British people of the need to overthrow capitalism and establish socialism. In part I believe this is due to the misconceptions of people's perception of the nature of the class system as it operates in the U.K. With the growing need to replace, renew and extend the housing stock in the 1950s that was destroyed in the war, together with the drive to increase exports in order to repay dept accrued as a consequence of the war, the unemployment of the pre-war period was largely eliminated.

However, among large elements of the so-called "blue collar workers", i.e. the industrial, engineering and building sectors, the perception arose that the "white collar workers", i.e. educational, administrative, retail and medical sectors, were somehow different. The blue collar workers regarded themselves, and were indeed regarded, as the "working class", whilst white collar workers were widely considered to be middle class. This perception was of course arrant nonsense since whilst blue collar workers were mostly hourly paid and large sections of white collar workers were salaried, they all equally relied on the provision of their labour, whether intellectual or physical, and frequently a combination of both, to an employer for a monetary reward in order to feed and house themselves and their families.

The failure to recognise this common bond among British people enabled, to a large extent, the continuation in power of the driving force that had established Capitalism in the 18th Century. This became apparent in 1952 when the Labour government, elected on a reform programme in 1945, despite its attempts to at least go some way to achieving what John Ball had said way back in the thirteen hundreds that "things will not be right in England until all is held in common". The establishment, alarmed at the potential likelihood of that objective, perhaps being achieved with the support of its cohorts abroad, sought to avoid that possibility and, with the active support of the media, there was increasing pressure generated to drive a wedge between blue and white collar workers which, throughout the 1960s and 1970s primarily took the form of attacks on the left, particularly in the Trades Union movement.

From all this pressure and propaganda emerged the eventual triumph of the establishment, with the election of Margaret Thatcher in 1979 who made a statement that "there is no such thing as society". From this, together with the promotion of rampant individualism and self seeking, has accrued all the current problems of countries throughout the world.

Margaret Thatcher has been followed by three Prime Ministers, not one of whom has done anything to expose or expunge the consequences of her philosophy. Yet the only way out of the mess we now find ourselves in was laid out quite clearly more than half a millennia ago when the rights of the common man were subsumed to the interests of the monarchy and its supporting elite. In its own interests, that elite moved the economic system from feudalism to capitalism yet, as the intellectuality of the common man increased, the vast majority of Britain's great inventors and innovators emerged from the common stock, not the elite!

The only true and successful ways in which humanity progresses and prospers is when the pressure for change comes from the bottom not the top. The situation that has developed in Britain since the late 1990s has been that of a patronising and condescending group of predominantly university educated, so-called professional, politicians that have emerged who allegedly seek to manage capitalism on behalf of the people as a whole. The incongruity of this aim is a further demonstration of the complete lack of political philosophy, ideology and understanding of the daily struggles of the common man. Not until the power to determine changes people want to achieve and the means by which they are achieved are placed in the hands of people as a whole and removed from the elite, elected or otherwise, can mankind truly progress.

The right of each to attain their full potential and use it to the benefit of the whole of mankind rather than self is the only way and must become our collective aim. From each according to their ability; to each according to their need.

FORWARD THE REVOLUTION.

Lightning Source UK Ltd.
Milton Keynes UK
UKOW021019050212

186702UK00001B/9/P